Integrated Early Childhood Behavioral Health in Primary Care

Rahil D. Briggs
Editor

Integrated Early Childhood Behavioral Health in Primary Care

A Guide to Implementation and Evaluation

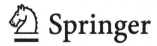 Springer

Editor
Rahil D. Briggs
Montefiore Health System
Bronx, NY, USA

ISBN 978-3-319-31813-4   ISBN 978-3-319-31815-8   (eBook)
DOI 10.1007/978-3-319-31815-8

Library of Congress Control Number: 2016940910

Printed on acid-free paper

This Springer imprint is published by Springer Nature
The registered company is Springer International Publishing AG Switzerland

Foreword

The practice of pediatrics emerged as a specialized domain of clinical medicine in the late nineteenth century. When the unique health needs of children were formalized through the establishment of the American Academy of Pediatrics in 1930, infection was the most prevalent threat to child survival, and infant feeding practices were a central focus of primary care. In the latter half of the twentieth century, developmental and behavioral difficulties constituted a growing percentage of the problems being brought to the primary care setting. Within this changing context, Richmond (1967) identified child development as the "basic science of pediatrics" and Haggerty, Roghmann, and Pless (1975) coined the term "new morbidities" to describe the seismic shift in parental concerns about their children's well-being.

As we now move through the second decade of the new millennium, increasing attention is being directed toward the adverse impacts of a host of social, behavioral, and economic threats to child health and development. As our recognition of these contextual factors has grown, our understanding of the critical influence of the child's environment of relationships has deepened. This expanding knowledge has generated increasingly greater demands for the pediatric primary care setting to address the immediate and long-term consequences of significant sources of ongoing stress, including poverty, racial and ethnic discrimination, maternal depression, parental substance abuse, and family and neighborhood violence, among many other disadvantages.

In 2012, the American Academy of Pediatrics issued a technical report (Shonkoff, Garner, The Committee on Psychosocial Aspects of Child and Family Health, Committee on Early Childhood, Adoption, and Dependent Care, & Section on Developmental and Behavioral Pediatrics, 2012) and an associated policy statement on toxic stress and the role of the pediatrician. The policy statement, which is cited frequently in this book, included the following bold statement: "Although the impact of these 'new' morbidities on pediatrics, public health, and society in general is no longer in question, the professional training and practice of pediatricians continues to focus primarily on the acute medical needs of individual children. The pressing question now confronting contemporary pediatrics is how we can have a greater impact on improving the life prospects of children and families who face these increasingly complex and persistent threats to healthy development" (American Academy of Pediatrics, Committee on Psychosocial Aspects of Child and Family Health, Committee on Early Childhood, Adoption, and Dependent Care, Section on Developmental and Behavioral Pediatrics, Garner, & Shonkoff, 2012).

The challenges presented by this changing context have stimulated the evolving development of the field that is the subject of this book—integrated early childhood behavioral health in primary care. As stated by Rahil Briggs at the end of the first chapter, this broader approach to health promotion and disease prevention for young children provides "much needed services in the only universally accessed and non-stigmatized setting we have for very young children." Its origins lie at the intersection of three complementary bodies of work that have generated growing attention over the past two decades. The first is the reported association between adverse childhood experiences (ACEs) and adult disease. The second is the concept of toxic stress, which refers to the physiological disruptions produced by excessive activation of stress response systems which can have a "wear-and-tear" effect on the brain and throughout the body. The third is the notion of trauma-informed care, which provides a framework for treating individuals who have had significant exposure to violence, loss, or other emotionally harmful experiences. Taken together, ACE scores quantify increased risk (but not a diagnosis) of health problems; toxic stress focuses on causal mechanisms that link adversity to impairments in learning, behavior, and health; and trauma-informed care provides guidelines for effective treatment. Building on their diverse origins in epidemiology, biology, and clinical practice, these three bodies of work inform an enhanced framework for pediatric primary care that is the focus of this important book.

Throughout this volume, Briggs and her colleagues provide a rich compendium of practical information about this evolving field of practice. The contributing authors bring different sets of lenses to a common agenda and share a wealth of lessons learned from their own experiences "on the ground." Beyond its immediate utility for the primary care community, this book also provides a valuable benchmark for current best practice as a starting point (not a final destination) for addressing contemporary health problems. With this latter goal in mind, advances in neuroscience, molecular biology, and epigenetics constitute a new basic science for pediatrics—and offer a rich resource for those readers who wish to push the leading edge of behavioral health even further and create a twenty-first century model of primary care for young children.

The Basic Science of Early Childhood Behavioral Health

Building on a well-established, multidisciplinary knowledge base that has been built over more than half a century, advances in the biological, behavioral, and social sciences have generated the following core concepts that currently constitute a credible basic science for guiding policies and programs focused on health promotion and disease prevention, as well as for informing early childhood behavioral health more specifically:

- Brains are built over time, and a substantial proportion is constructed during the early years of life. The architecture of the developing brain is built through an ongoing process that begins before birth, continues into adulthood, and establishes either a sturdy or a fragile foundation for a lifetime of health, learning, and behavior.
- The interaction of genes and experiences shapes the circuitry of the developing brain. Scientists have discovered that the experiences children have early in life—and the environments in which they live—not only shape their developing brain architecture but also affect how genes are turned on and off and even whether some are expressed at all.
- Children develop in an environment of relationships that begins in the family but also involves other adults who play important roles in their lives, such as providers of early care and education, extended family members, physicians, nurses, social workers, coaches, and neighbors. These relationships affect virtually all aspects of development—intellectual, social, emotional, physical, and behavioral.
- Skill begets skill as brains are built in a hierarchical fashion from the bottom up, with increasingly complex circuits building on simpler circuits and increasingly complex and adaptive skills emerging with age. Times of exceptional sensitivity to the effects of experiences on different brain circuits are called *critical* or *sensitive periods*. These periods begin and end at different ages for different parts of the brain.
- Cognitive, emotional, and social capacities are inextricably intertwined in the architecture of the brain, and the circuitry that affects learning and behavior is interconnected with physiological systems that affect health. The brain is a highly integrated organ and its many functions operate in a richly coordinated fashion. All human capabilities and both physical and mental well-being develop through a lifelong process that is deeply embedded in the function of the brain, cardiovascular, immune, neuroendocrine, and metabolic systems.
- Research on the biology of stress shows how major adversity, such as extreme poverty, abuse, or neglect, can "get under the skin" and result in physiological disruptions that affect lifelong outcomes in learning, behavior, and health. This rapidly advancing science can help us identify preventive measures to avoid these negative effects and can inform more intensive treatment options to counterbalance the problems that are caused by early and more severe adversity.
- Toxic stress responses can lead to lifelong impairments in health and development. Learning how to cope with adversity is an important part of healthy child development. When a young child's stress response systems are activated within an environment of supportive adult relationships, the responses are either positive or tolerable, and the result is the development of a well-functioning stress response system. When the stress response is activated continually or triggered repeatedly by multiple threats in the absence of adult support, it can be toxic and have a cumulative toll on a child's physical and mental health for a lifetime.

- Problems in cognitive, social, and emotional development, as well as impairments in physical and mental health, often result from complex interactions between a child's genetic predisposition and his or her exposure to significant adversity. These kinds of interactions early in life can prime neurobiological stress systems to become hyperresponsive to adversity. This response can create an unstable foundation for development in general, and for physical and mental health specifically, that endures well into the adult years.
- Brain plasticity and the ability to change behavior decrease over time because the increasing specialization of the maturing brain makes it both more efficient and less capable of reorganizing and adapting to new or unanticipated challenges. Although windows of opportunity for skill development and behavioral adaptation remain open for many years, trying to change behavior or build new skills on a foundation of brain circuits that were not wired properly when they were first formed requires more work for both individuals and society.
- Positive early experiences, consistent support from adults, and the development of adaptive skills can counterbalance adversity and build resilience. The connection between adverse early life experiences and a wide range of costly social problems, such as poor school achievement, low economic productivity, criminal behavior, and impaired health, is well documented. Understanding why some people develop the adaptive capacities to overcome significant disadvantage while others do not is key to enabling more children to experience positive outcomes and build a more resilient society.

Current Best Practices and the Future of Behavioral Health in Primary Care

Because developmental and behavioral problems in childhood can have lifelong effects on both physical and mental health, addressing these concerns early in life is a fundamental pediatric responsibility. The principles and practices described in this volume represent an important leading edge in the delivery of primary healthcare—and this book serves as a valuable resource for a range of disciplines involved in services for young children and their families as well as in training the professionals who deliver those services.

The challenges facing integrated early childhood behavioral health in the primary care setting mirror the challenges that have confronted the broader field of early childhood policy and practice for half a century—from child care and early education to family support programs and child welfare services, among many others. On the positive side, multiple interventions have been developed to address the origins of disparities in early development and later school achievement, and extensive program evaluation research has documented both positive impacts for many program participants and strong economic returns for society. Without minimizing the importance of these documented benefits, however, it is essential that we acknowledge that the quality of implementation when programs are taken to scale is highly variable, the magnitude of effects typically falls within the small to moderate range, and long-term sustainability of short-term gains has been difficult to achieve. Unlocking the answers to these challenges and producing breakthrough outcomes require that we apply new insights from both cutting-edge science and the kind of practical, on-the-ground experience catalogued in this book (Shonkoff & Fisher, 2013).

The full promise of an integrated approach to behavioral health in primary care practice lies in the considerable work that remains to be done if we truly want to transform the lives (and future life prospects) of children and families facing significant adversity. That quest begins with the simple yet powerful recognition that effective interventions require resources and expertise that match the challenges they are asked to address—and different precipitants of toxic stress often require different responses from a variety of systems. Achieving greater understanding of variations in susceptibility to adversity and determining the appropriate mix of strategies to capitalize on existing strengths and address unmet needs are critical challenges that must be addressed.

The general question of whether a specific intervention "works" *on average* has guided early childhood policy and practice for decades. In order for integrated behavioral health to achieve greater impacts in the context of primary healthcare, it is essential that leaders in the field begin to focus more explicitly on two critical questions. First, what kinds of concerns in what kinds of children and families are benefitting the most (and why) from specific practices that are being implemented in the pediatric setting? Second, and equally important, what kinds of problems in what kinds of contexts are responding the least or not at all—and why? Identifying the former will provide a powerful knowledge base for replication and targeted scaling that will drive the growth of this important field. Focusing on the latter must stimulate a search for new intervention strategies that draws on the collective insights, expertise, and experiences of practitioners, researchers, program developers, and parents whose children's needs are not being fully met. In the final analysis, significantly larger impacts will be achieved for larger numbers of children and families if advances in scientific knowledge are leveraged to drive the design, testing, and scaling of a diversified portfolio of well-defined services that are matched to available resources, identified needs, and specific outcomes for different groups of children and families.

One additional piece of the impact evaluation puzzle that must be put into place to complete the story presented throughout this volume is the need to raise the bar on goals and expectations for integrated behavioral health for young children. The wealth of baseline information derived from two decades of implementation and evaluation of the Healthy Steps program provides a useful place to begin this task. As described in this book, an expanded and more vigorous approach to screening and intervention within a relationship-based model of primary healthcare can produce a wide range of impacts on parents' knowledge about child development, child-rearing practices in the home, and short-term effects on reported child behaviors.

In addition, participating families reported high levels of satisfaction with the services they received and they engaged more consistently with their child's pediatric practice. What remains to be done is a more segmented approach to assessing impacts on two key objectives—what kinds of concerns and needs are served well by the current service model and what kinds of problems require far more effort and specialized expertise than the pediatric primary care setting can be expected to provide? This need for greater differentiation among children and families facing adversity is arguably one of the most important challenges facing the field—and it is unquestionably the most important challenge facing those who seek to serve children and families who are bearing the greatest burdens of disadvantage in the earliest years of life.

Finally, it is clear that the early childhood origins of impairments in learning, behavior, and health often lie beyond the walls of the medical office or hospital setting. Indeed, for many young children, the boundaries of pediatric concern must move beyond the domain of medical services and expand into the larger ecology of the community, state, and society. Although the responsibility for these larger and exceedingly more complex challenges does not rest solely on those healthcare providers who are focusing on the integration of behavioral health expertise into primary care, the leading edge of this important field offers a vital source of expertise and experience to fuel fresh thinking and new ideas. Briggs and her colleagues have produced a book that provides an important starting point for taking on this challenge. The time is long overdue for the entire pediatric community to join in this journey.

Cambridge, MA, USA   Jack P. Shonkoff, M.D.
Julius B. Richmond FAMRI Professor
of Child Health and Development
Harvard T.H. Chan School of Public Health
and Harvard Graduate School of Education
Harvard University

References

American Academy of Pediatrics, Committee on Psychosocial Aspects of Child and Family Health, Committee on Early Childhood, Adoption, and Dependent Care, Section on Developmental and Behavioral Pediatrics, Garner, A. S., & Shonkoff, J. P. (2012). Early childhood adversity, toxic stress, and the role of the pediatrician: Translating developmental science into lifelong health. *Pediatrics, 129*(1), e224–e231.

Haggerty, R. J., Roghman, R. K., & Pless, I. B. (1975). *Child health and the community*. New York, NY: Wiley.

Richmond, J. (1967). Child development: A basic science for pediatrics. *Pediatrics, 39*, 649–658.

Shonkoff, J., & Fisher, P. (2013). Rethinking evidence-based practice and two-generation programs to create the future of early childhood policy. *Development and Psychopathology, 25*, 1635–1653.

Shonkoff, J. P., Garner, A. S., The Committee on Psychosocial Aspects of Child and Family Health, Committee on Early Childhood, Adoption, and Dependent Care, & Section on Developmental and Behavioral Pediatrics. (2012). The lifelong effects of early childhood adversity and toxic stress. *Pediatrics, 129*(1), e232–e246.

Acknowledgments

Dr. Briggs wishes to acknowledge the patients and families who guide our work, motivate us to improve our models of care, and remind us of the importance of getting it right, for generations present and future.

Contents

About the Editor

Rahil D. Briggs Psy.D. is associate professor of pediatrics at Albert Einstein College of Medicine, director of Healthy Steps at Montefiore, and the director of Pediatric Behavioral Health Services at Montefiore Medical Group. Dr. Briggs joined Einstein and Montefiore in 2005 as the director and founder of Healthy Steps at Montefiore. She was appointed assistant professor of pediatrics in 2008 and expanded the Healthy Steps program to multiple sites within Montefiore Medical Group in 2009 and 2013. She was named the director of Pediatric Behavioral Health Services at Montefiore in 2013 to spearhead the formation of one of the most comprehensive integrated pediatric behavioral health systems in the nation. Her work concentrates on co-location of mental health specialists within primary care pediatrics, with a focus on prevention, early childhood mental health and development, and parent–child relationships. Dr. Briggs completed her undergraduate work at Duke University (magna cum laude) and her doctoral work at New York University.

Contributors

Brooke Allman Rose F. Kennedy Children's Evaluation and Rehabilitation Center, Montefiore Medical Center, Bronx, NY, USA

Diane Bloomfield Division of Academic General Pediatrics, Children's Hospital at Montefiore, Albert Einstein College of Medicine, Bronx, NY, USA

Rahil D. Briggs Montefiore Health System, Bronx, NY, USA

Nicole Brown Division of Academic General Pediatrics, Children's Hospital at Montefiore, Albert Einstein College of Medicine, Bronx, NY, USA

Melissa Buchholz University of Colorado School of Medicine, Children's Hospital Colorado, Aurora, CO, USA

Rosy Chhabra Albert Einstein College of Medicine, Bronx, NY, USA

Dana E. Crawford Montefiore Health System, Bronx, NY, USA

Kate Cuno Montefiore Health System, Bronx, NY, USA

Shanta Rishi Dube Georgia State University, Atlanta, GA, USA

Helena Duch Columbia University, Mailman School of Public Health, New York, NY, USA

Miguelina Germán Montefiore Health System, Bronx, NY, USA

Rebecca Schrag Hershberg Montefiore Health System, Bronx, NY, USA

Margot Kaplan-Sanoff Healthy Steps, Zero to Three, Washington, DC, USA

Theodore Kastner Rose F. Kennedy Children's Evaluation and Rehabilitation Center, Montefiore Medical Center, Bronx, NY, USA

Laura Krug Montefiore Health System, Bronx, NY, USA

Anne Murphy Rose F. Kennedy Children's Evaluation and Rehabilitation Center, Montefiore Medical Center, Bronx, NY, USA

Emily F. Muther University of Colorado School of Medicine, Children's Hospital Colorado, Aurora, CO, USA

Andrew D. Racine Montefiore Medicine, Bronx, NY, USA

Ellen Johnson Silver Albert Einstein College of Medicine, Bronx, NY, USA

Howard Steele New School for Social Research, New York, NY, USA

Miriam Steele New School for Social Research, New York, NY, USA

Ayelet Talmi University of Colorado School of Medicine, Children's Hospital Colorado, Aurora, CO, USA

Polina Umylny Montefiore Health System, Bronx, NY, USA

Karen Warman Division of Academic General Pediatrics, Children's Hospital at Montefiore, Albert Einstein College of Medicine, Bronx, NY, USA

Chapter 1
Introduction

Rahil D. Briggs

The field of integrated early childhood behavioral health in primary care has been slowly moving forward for the last 20 years or so, and now feels poised to truly expand to scale. The vast scientific breakthroughs of the last decades, along with a new understanding of the importance of integrated healthcare, the need for prevention of toxic stress, and the power of trauma informed care, have paved the way for an exciting and well-deserved expansion of the movement. As a society, if we seek a better set of outcomes related to education, prosperity, and health and wellness, we must focus our attention on the uniquely transformative platform of integrated early childhood behavioral health within primary care. Primary care is the one system we have that provides an opportunity to gauge the progress of all our young children and families. With integrated early childhood behavioral health providers alongside primary care practitioners, focused on the young child and his or her caregivers together in a two-generation model, we have the opportunity to practice true, population based prevention and help ensure the next generation has the strongest start yet.

We offer this volume to briefly help reiterate the basis for integrated early childhood behavioral health in primary care, but more notably to focus primarily on the most important questions of "how/what." Any time that a model of clinical service delivery expands, multiple questions arise. Most often, the "why" of the matter has essentially been resolved. That is, the field has determined that such an expansion is justified to address the problem at hand. Although there are always late adopters, the bulk of the field is seeking to answer the next set of questions, the "how/what." A misstep during the how/what phase of expansion may be particularly concerning, as the momentum can stall just as soon as it began.

Before we outline the contents of the volume, some guiding definitions may be helpful. We have attempted to align ourselves with the original volume regarding adult integrated behavioral healthcare, edited by Hunter and colleagues and focused

R.D. Briggs, Psy.D (✉)
Montefiore Health System, Bronx, NY, USA
e-mail: rabriggs@montefiore.org

© Springer International Publishing Switzerland 2016
R.D. Briggs (ed.), *Integrated Early Childhood Behavioral Health
in Primary Care*, DOI 10.1007/978-3-319-31815-8_1

exclusively on the provision of integrated behavioral healthcare services in the adult primary care setting (Hunter, Goodie, Oordt, & Dobmeyer, 2009). Therein, they provide a comprehensive description of the continuum of care between collaborative, co-located, and integrated. They note that collaborative care often refers to agreements between providers, working in separate systems and facilities, to exchange information about shared patients. Co-located care takes that relationship a bit further and often has those same providers, still employed by separate systems, but now working alongside each other in a shared facility. Finally, integrated care is provided by a team of providers, employed and working in the same system, using one treatment plan, a shared medical record, and truly functioning as a patient care team.

The other area to define is what we mean by "early childhood" when referring to programs and providers. While one chapter in this volume describes the workforce issue at length, and another describes various programs, we generally refer to the "early childhood" period as anything starting either prenatally or around the birth of the child, and depending on resources, it may extend through child age 3, 5, or even 8. Finally, we note that "pediatric practice" refers to any medical professional caring for children, including Family Medicine and Nurse Practitioner colleagues.

In this volume, we review questions of program design and workforce development, discuss issues of evaluation and financial sustainability, and share our extensive lessons learned via reports from early childhood behavioral health and pediatric providers with experience in these models of care. We provide "on the ground" examples whenever possible to illustrate real world application of the topics presented, and create a tone less theoretical and more pragmatic where possible.

The organization of the volume was driven by the significant number of requests for consultation received since we started our integrated early childhood programming over 10 years ago. In increasing numbers, we have received multiple calls and e-mails, first every few months and more recently on a weekly basis. Other hospital systems and community mental health agencies have wanted to know everything from program design to staffing ratios, as they seek to move into this exciting new field. We hope this volume helps answer many of the questions from our colleagues, and spreads the answers more quickly than possible during individual calls and meetings. Let the revolution in integrated early childhood behavioral health programming begin!

The first section of the book features chapters focused on two important aspects of the "why" that we believe bear emphasis. We do not attempt to comprehensively review the scientific rationale behind addressing early childhood behavioral health, as that has been done quite succinctly by Shonkoff and colleagues, referred to in the foreword of this volume. Instead, we focus first on Adverse Childhood Experiences (ACEs)/trauma informed care and, second, on return on investment (ROI) and cost-effectiveness evaluations. In the proverbial three legged stool of helping healthcare systems get behind integrated early childhood behavioral health with real dollars and commitment, the brain science is critical, but should be augmented by the long-term health outcomes of the ACEs research and the cost-effectiveness of early childhood programming.

To begin, Murphy et al. address the American Academy of Pediatrics' policy statement on the need to address toxic stress within primary care pediatrics. Building on the vast legacy of ACEs literature, and their own unique innovations around

ACEs, Dr. Murphy and colleagues paint a compelling picture of the power of the intergenerational transmission of trauma, and the ways in which an integrated primary care practice might address this critical public health issue. Rather than a unique, isolated phenomenon, the authors demonstrate that ACEs are in fact a common occurrence, have a large impact on parental functioning, and are a key target of intervention in this arena. Although some pediatric practices have waded into the ACEs waters, there is still significant apprehension around addressing ACEs in primary care, despite the powerful reasons to do so. The chapter highlights four commonly heard concerns: provider discomfort around ACEs, perceived misalignment between asking parents about their own childhood during a pediatric visit, the responsibility of mandated reporting regarding ACEs, and the need for follow-up care upon discovery of ACEs. In each area of concern, the authors provide rich experience-based responses to facilitate integration of ACEs and trauma informed care into primary care pediatrics, particularly focused on the early childhood domain and the parent–child relationship.

The second chapter in this section addresses the remarkable ROI when we intervene early, and the reasons to do so from an economics perspective. Via application of human capital theory to the arena of early childhood development/behavior, Andrew Racine paints a sophisticated picture of the interplay between these two fields. Dr. Racine is uniquely qualified to address this topic, as both a pediatrician and an economist, and helps outline the empirical findings related to economic evaluations of early childhood programs. Although most readers will be familiar with the usual suspects of ROI in early childhood (Perry Preschool, Abecedarian, etc.), the chapter goes beyond a summary of these findings to identify important considerations in conducting future cost-effectiveness evaluations that can potentially be applied to a wide range of integrated early childhood behavioral health programs. Finally, the chapter concludes with policy implications, noting the limit of relying simply on economic markets to encourage programming. Dr. Racine suggests that the "illumination of the neurological and molecular biological mechanisms influencing the developing brain, coupled with an accumulation of persuasive empirical evidence regarding the economic benefits of investing in early child development, is shifting social perception toward an acknowledgment that the time has come to redefine public responsibility toward fostering the human capital stock of the next generation of citizens."

From a brief foray into the "why," we move to the most substantial part of the volume, the "how/what," comprising seven chapters that aim to guide anyone— from practitioners to policy makers—through the various important design considerations that play a role in the creation and implementation of integrated early childhood behavioral health programs.

We begin with an attempt to quantify the "goodness of fit" between the major evidence based early childhood behavioral health interventions and primary care. This chapter was written by Crawford and Briggs in recognition that, simply because a program has an evidence base in one setting, it does not mean it will necessarily be a good fit within another setting. Primary care is a unique venue, and families interface with primary care differently than they might a mental health clinic or other locale. For example, primary care treatment is episodic and needs-based, rather than divided into weekly sessions scheduled in advance, as might be the case in a behavioral health clinic. Furthermore, the primary care environment is a fast paced, multidisciplinary setting focused on improving care while reducing costs. Thus, long-term treatments, or programs that are especially costly to implement, may not be ideal or, even, appropriate. This chapter focuses on seven points we deem critical when determining the goodness of fit between a particular program and primary care and concludes with programmatic recommendations for early childhood integrated care.

Next, Kaplan-Sanoff and Briggs describe The Healthy Steps program, the original early childhood evidence based intervention specifically designed for integration into primary care settings, including the history, the cornerstones of the intervention model, lessons learned, and challenges encountered during the replication phase. The chapter closes with a look toward the future, as Healthy Steps has recently (2015) joined forces with ZERO TO THREE, which has secured funding to examine effective replication, sustainability, and scalability pathways for the Healthy Steps model. The goal is to build the capacity and infrastructure of the National Healthy Steps Office at ZERO TO THREE to design a blueprint for the next stage of growth and evaluation.

The second part of this "what/how" section focuses on workforce development/training, challenges in integration and the silos that resist change, the need to focus on culturally relevant interventions, and reimbursement and evaluation of programs.

To begin, Hershberg and Briggs discuss the workforce development and training needs for providers of early childhood behavioral healthcare in an integrated setting. We first address the unique tasks and requirements of the job, and the skills and abilities that are needed to do the work most effectively. We then explore the goodness of fit between certain fields of study (such as social work, nursing, and psychology) and integrated early childhood behavioral healthcare. We look at the qualities and traits needed in order to function successfully in primary care, and argue that successful practitioners will focus on both provision of patient care *and* culture and practice change, and we conclude with a focus on the need for continual training and ongoing focus on quality.

The idea of culture and practice change is a salient one for effective wide scale provision of integrated early childhood behavioral health programming. Briggs, Germán, and Hershberg discuss issues of silos and integration challenges via a review of our decade of integrated early childhood behavioral healthcare experience at Montefiore Medical Center in the Bronx, NY. Constantly infusing lessons learned and reasons for programming decisions, we present our current program model (including setting, population served, and design). We discuss our use of universal ACEs screening to best identify families who might benefit from our services, and review the many steps and mistakes made along our journey toward arriving at this design. We review our universal screening schedule for young children and their caregivers and present our two tracks of intervention: intensive services for those families most at risk, and short-term behavior and development consultations for the general population. We also discuss our unique parental mental health programming, and the benefits of providing treatment for parents within the pediatric setting.

To close, we summarize our major lessons learned: how to break down silos while respecting the hierarchy implicit in medical settings, how to balance documentation and privacy concerns within an integrated setting, and the need to combat isolation amongst providers in this field, who are often surrounded by medical professionals and lack behavioral health colleagues on-site.

The next chapter (Duch, Germán and Cuno) discusses the important cultural variability that impacts child–parent relationships, norms, and expectations around early childhood development, and thus the role of the culturally competent early childhood behavioral health provider within a pediatric setting. Although we recognize that a single chapter on this topic is insufficient (there could be a volume unto itself), we nonetheless believe so wholeheartedly in its importance that we determined some attention was far better than none. The authors conducted a comprehensive review of the literature and summarize the major findings related to cultural norms and differences within three very common arenas of early childhood behavioral health consultations: discipline, feeding, and sleep. They combine this with a sensitive nod toward the difference between simple cultural competence and culturally competent *care*, as per the American Academy of Pediatrics guidelines. Via inclusion of multiple on the ground examples, the authors conclude with five recommendations to ensure careful consideration of parenting differences within practice, regardless of the potential match or mismatch between provider and patient.

Program financing and evaluation round out this "what/how" section, as necessary and critical aspects of any successful integrated early childhood behavioral health program. Talmi and colleagues outline the current healthcare funding landscape (which has certainly changed by the time of publication, reflecting the rapidly changing context), describe on the ground examples to develop and financially sustain integrated behavioral health programming, and conclude with recommendations and strategies for integrated early childhood services. They present a compelling framework of the "Four Ps" of financial sustainability: procedures, practice, payment, and policy. Within this framework, the authors discuss service delivery and billing models, grant funding potentials, and conclude with policy recommendations to ensure long-term viability of integrated early childhood behavioral health programs.

An oft neglected, yet critically important aspect of effective programming is evaluation. Silver and Chhabra, with decades of evaluation experience between them, outline the reasons for evaluation, and the unique considerations depending on the audience for the evaluation results. They present five considerations for developing the focus of an evaluation, discuss formative versus summative evaluation, and guide the reader through a measures selection framework. Finally, the authors present an on the ground example of a very simple yet important evaluation, that of measuring patient satisfaction.

Although we have infused on the ground examples throughout the chapters, the volume concludes with more in-depth personal perspectives on integrated care, from the points of view of both pediatric and early childhood behavioral health providers. Pediatricians Brown, Bloomfield, and Warman present their experience as part of the Montefiore Healthy Steps program. From their perspective, they offer guidelines for implementation of screening, educational programming, and shared care that can work within a busy urban pediatric setting. After addressing the real concerns regarding time demands and changes in role definition, they note the particular benefits of integrated early childhood behavioral health programming, including increased continuity of care, enhanced provision of social supports, and improved delivery of family centered care. They note both individual and practice transformation, as a result of sharing their patients with the Healthy Steps Specialists in their practice sites.

The volume closes with the voices of two clinicians who have provided care to thousands of children and families within the Montefiore Healthy Steps program. Krug and Umlyny, two senior Healthy Steps Specialists, present cases that are representative of our typical families. First, they present a mother of four, at the pediatric practice for her infant's 1 month checkup. This 1 month old was born prematurely, and was living with her mother and three siblings in transitional housing. This case presented opportunities to work with a medically fragile child, a parent with misconceived notions regarding spoiling an infant, the parent–child relationships with older children that often suffer due to the arrival of a new baby, and the impact of parental trauma (assessed via ACEs) on her perceptions of her children's behaviors. The second family presented is a short-term behavior and development consultation, for a 3 year old with tantrums and aggression. In just three sessions, the early childhood behavioral health specialist was able to reassure parents who were convinced their child had a diagnosable disorder, such as Attention Deficit Hyperactivity Disorder (ADHD), and provide them with strategies to encourage improved behavior and social emotional development in their son. The final case example describes our parental mental health services, focused on a young mother who was experiencing panic attacks. Fearful of leaving the house, and thus concerned that she might lose her job, this mother received integrated care from the Healthy Steps Specialist and the integrated psychiatrist, and was quickly able to resume her regular activities.

Integrated early childhood behavioral healthcare is poised to transform the early childhood landscape and to provide much needed services in the only universally accessed and non-stigmatized setting we have for very young children. The possibilities are significant and we hope that this volume will guide the reader through potential questions of implementation and evaluation. The momentum is here, and we must proceed quickly yet carefully to ensure high quality early childhood integrated behavioral health programming. The future depends on it.

Reference

Hunter, C. L., Goodie, J. L., Oordt, M. S., & Dobmeyer, A. C. (Eds.). (2009). *Integrated behavioral health in primary care: Step-by-step guidance for assessment and intervention.* Washington, DC: American Psychological Association.

Chapter 2
The Clinical Adverse Childhood Experiences (ACEs) Questionnaire: Implications for Trauma-Informed Behavioral Healthcare

Anne Murphy, Howard Steele, Miriam Steele, Brooke Allman, Theodore Kastner, and Shanta Rishi Dube

Abstract Within primary care pediatrics, there is an optimal and essential opportunity to educate parents on how the pernicious effects of toxic stress have impacted their lives and how they can prevent and/or buffer the effects of stress in their child's life. The recommendation from the 2012 American Academy of Pediatrics policy statement is to infuse a trauma-informed perspective into pediatrics, and this may be accomplished by introducing providers to the Adverse Childhood Experiences (ACEs) Study and the essential role of two-generational ACE screening. The seminal ACEs studies provided a paradigm shift in our understanding of the impact of childhood trauma on both physical and mental health throughout the life span. At the same time, the intergenerational link between childhood experiences and quality of parenting has been well established in attachment research. Integrating these two bodies of work has led to new ways of understanding the links between parental experiences in their own childhood and the quality of the parent–child relationship with their offspring. The link between trauma and attachment research provides a solid rationale for including the ACE measures into comprehensive screening and treatment with vulnerable families, many of whom regularly present to primary care pediatrics.

Keywords Adverse Childhood Experiences • Pediatric screening • Behavioral health • Parenting

---

A. Murphy, Ph.D. (✉) • B. Allman, L.C.S.W. • T. Kastner, M.D.
Rose F. Kennedy Children's Evaluation and Rehabilitation Center,
Montefiore Medical Center, Bronx, NY, USA
e-mail: amurphy1@montefiore.org; ballman@montefiore.org; tkastner@montefiore.org

H. Steele, Ph.D. • M. Steele, Ph.D.
New School for Social Research, New York, NY, USA
e-mail: steeleh@newschool.edu; steelem@newschool.edu

S.R. Dube, Ph.D., M.P.H.
Georgia State University, Atlanta, GA, USA
e-mail: sdube2@gsu.edu

© Springer International Publishing Switzerland 2016
R.D. Briggs (ed.), *Integrated Early Childhood Behavioral Health in Primary Care*, DOI 10.1007/978-3-319-31815-8_2

Introduction

In 2012, the American Academy of Pediatrics released a policy statement, which translated evidence from developmental science and created a sound basis for its indisputable recommendations on the need to address toxic stress within primary care pediatrics. This comprehensive mandate suggests that the pediatric community employs an ecobiodevelopmental (EBD) framework to conceptualize the social, behavioral, and economic determinants of lifelong disparities in physical and mental health. The EBD framework should guide pediatric training for current and future physicians, increasing awareness of the growing science that links childhood toxic stress with disruptions of the developing nervous, cardiovascular, immune, and metabolic systems, and the evidence that these disruptions can lead to lifelong impairments in learning, behavior, and physical/mental health. Additionally, the policy statement calls for the pediatric community to advocate for the development and implementation of new, evidence-based interventions that reduce sources of toxic stress and/or mitigate their adverse effects on young children. This might be accomplished by screening for toxic stress, educating parents on how to support children's emerging social-emotional-linguistic skills, and/or encouraging positive parenting techniques. However, the statement also suggests the necessity of developing and securing funding for children at risk beyond the medical home, and identifying and collaborating with local services that address risks of toxic stress.

Within primary care pediatrics, there is an optimal and essential opportunity to educate parents on how the pernicious effects of toxic stress have impacted their lives and how they can prevent and/or buffer the effects of stress in their child's life. Practically speaking, one valuable vehicle to operationalize the policy statement's recommendations is to infuse a trauma-informed perspective into pediatrics by introducing providers to the Adverse Childhood Experiences Study and the essential role of two-generational ACE screening.

The seminal Adverse Childhood Experiences (ACEs) studies (Dube et al., 2003; Felitti et al., 1998) provided a paradigm shift in our understanding of the impact of childhood trauma on both physical and mental health throughout the life span. At the same time, the intergenerational link between childhood experiences and quality of parenting has been well established in the attachment research literature (Bowlby, 1969, 1982, 1988; Main, Hesse, & Goldwyn, 2008; Pederson, Gleason, Moran, & Bento, 1998; van IJzendoorn, 1995; Ward & Carlson, 1995). Integrating these two bodies of work has led to new ways of understanding the links between parental experiences in their own childhood and the quality of the parent–child relationship with their offspring (Murphy et al., 2014). The link between trauma and attachment research provides a solid rationale for including the ACE measures into comprehensive screening and treatment with vulnerable families, many of whom regularly present to primary care pediatrics. This chapter will discuss the implications of high ACEs on parenting, how to integrate ACEs screening into pediatric settings, and the use of ACEs in trauma-informed intervention.

The Adverse Childhood Experiences Study

In 1995, Kaiser Permanente in Southern California and the Centers for Disease Control and Prevention (CDC) collaborated on a large-scale epidemiologic investigation, the Adverse Childhood Experiences (ACE) Study. The ACE Study included a cohort of over 17,000 adult health maintenance organization (HMO) members and retrospectively assessed exposures to childhood stressors, such as physical, emotional and sexual abuse, emotional and physical neglect, household substance abuse and mental illness, parental discord, witnessing domestic violence, and criminality in the home. The assessment of these ten ACEs was a significant departure from existing research in the field, which tended to examine the contribution of *single* forms of abuse with health outcomes. In taking this novel approach, the ACE Study was one of the first epidemiologic studies to not only demonstrate that exposures to each of the ten categories of childhood abuse, neglect, and family dysfunction are common, but that they are highly interrelated (Dube et al., 2003; Dube, Anda, Felitti, Edwards, & Croft, 2002; Felitti et al., 1998). Using the total number of reported ACEs, or ACE score, research from the ACE Study has documented that close to two-thirds of the adult cohort reported experiencing at least one ACE, and 40 % reported two or more.

The ACE study also demonstrated that abuse, neglect, and serious forms of household dysfunction are associated with multiple social, physical, behavioral, and mental health problems that emerge in adolescence and persist into adulthood. For example, each childhood exposure was associated with an elevated risk of smoking, illicit drug use, alcohol abuse, suicidality, and depression (Anda et al., 1999; Chapman et al., 2004; Dube et al., 2003, 2006, 2009; Dube, Cook, & Edwards, 2010; Felitti et al., 1998). Exposure to abuse, neglect, and serious household dysfunction were found to be associated with specific medical and physical health outcomes, including autoimmune disorders, cardiovascular disease, and liver disease (Dube et al., 2009; Felitti et al., 1998). Most importantly, the ACE study has documented that the childhood adversities studied tend to co-occur, and there was a strong graded dose–response relationship between the ACE score and all of the aforementioned behavioral, social, and health outcomes (Dube et al., 2001, 2002, 2003; Felitti et al., 1998; Harris, Putman, & Fairbank, 2004).

The ACE study findings have shown that exposure to childhood abuse and other forms of trauma likely activates the stress response, potentially disrupting the developing nervous, immune, and metabolic systems of children, and thereby providing biological plausibility for epidemiological findings (De Bellis et al., 1999; Hair, Hanson, Wolfe, & Pollak, 2015; Lehman, Taylor, Kiefe, & Seeman, 2009; Stein, Koverola, Hanna, Torchia, & McClarty, 1997; Teicher et al., 1997). These insights into childhood determinants of adverse health outcomes throughout the life span, provided in the ACE study and other similar studies, suggest the need for two generation behavioral health interventions, delivered in a prevention context, beginning as early as possible and focused on the parent–child dyad.

ACEs and Parenting: The Intergenerational Transmission of Risk

While previous research from the ACE study has demonstrated the long-term health impact of numerous stressful and traumatic childhood exposures, as summarized above, there is less appreciation of the pernicious impact of exposure to ACEs (in the first 18 years of life) and adult functioning in the parental role. Some of the outcomes demonstrated to be associated with ACEs most certainly tax a parent's ability to provide sensitive and responsive care to the next generation, and detract from one's ability to successfully embrace the parental role. These include depression (Chapman et al., 2004), suicidality (Dube et al., 2001), risk of illicit drug use, HIV, sexual risk behavior (Dube et al., 2003; Meade, Kershaw, Hansen, & Sikkema, 2009), and alcohol abuse (Dube, Anda, et al., 2001; Dube et al., 2002, 2005). Additionally, high levels of ACEs are associated with parenting stress (Steele et al., 2016) and the absence of secure adult attachment classifications (Murphy, et al., 2014) on the Adult Attachment Interview (AAI) (Main, Goldwyn, & Hesse, 2003). This is important, as the AAI is the gold standard measure of attachment patterns (Main et al., 2003, 2008; Main, Kaplan, & Cassidy, 1985) in adults and a robust predictor of attachment in the next generation of parent–child attachment relationships, thus indicating the significant potential for pronounced difficulties in parenting and parent–child relationship difficulties based on parental ACEs.

Murphy et al.'s (2014) study on the impact of ACEs and attachment provides a better understanding of the mechanisms through which problematic parenting may occur. This research found that mothers who reported four or more ACEs demonstrated significantly higher rates of unresolved loss or trauma in response to the AAI. Interviews classified as Unresolved with regard to loss and/or trauma predict the most troubling infant–parent relationships, in which fear and disorganization predominate (Lyons-Ruth & Jacobvitz, 2008; Steele, Steele, & Fonagy, 1996; van IJzendoorn, 1995). Parents who are unable to make sense of their own traumatic childhood experiences are at increased risk of bringing these unresolved problems into their relationships with their own children, resulting in Disorganized attachment, the most concerning parent–child attachment classification. Children who are classified as Disorganized are more likely to exhibit internalizing (Groh et al., 2014) and externalizing behavior problems (Belsky & Fearon, 2002; Lyons-Ruth & Jacobvitz, 2008) later in childhood, and to suffer from dissociation and personality disorders in late adolescence and young adulthood (Lyons-Ruth & Jacobvitz, 2008). These findings suggest the need for bringing the discussion of the implications of high ACEs on parenting (Murphy et al., 2014) into primary pediatric and clinical settings (Dube et al., 2003).

Adverse Childhood Experiences and Healthcare Reform

As the USA works to achieve high value healthcare, we must pursue a broad range of linked goals. These goals are referred to as the "Triple Aim," and include improving the individual experience of care, improving the health of populations, and reducing the per capita costs of care for populations (Berwick, Nolan, & Whittington, 2008). Trauma-informed care includes attention to preventing ACEs in addition to treating ACEs in parents and in their children. To describe the impact of trauma, and especially multiple traumas, Bessel Van der Kolk (1994) coined the phrase, "the body keeps score."

On the Ground Example

For example, New York State Medicaid redesign efforts to develop Children's Health Homes (CHH) incorporate the use of trauma-informed assessments, often including ACE scores, to help determine acuity levels https://www.health.ny.gov/health_care/medicaid/program/medicaid:health_homes/docs/cans_0_5.pdf. Children with histories of ACEs will be identified as experiencing a qualifying factor, as it is well documented that these children are often medically complex, and are thus often high users of medical services.

In addition to the physical costs of ACEs throughout the life span, there are also financial costs in terms of the immediate and long-term cumulative price of maltreatment, which has been well documented by economists (Heckman, 2006). The economic burden of ACEs includes not only the immediate health and social welfare costs for children exposed to abuse, neglect, and serious family dysfunction, but also the long-term health and social costs for the survivors of abuse and neglect. The relevance of the economic costs of ACEs further underscores the need to reduce or prevent the occurrence of ACEs, and the universally accessed pediatric primary care environment may be the best venue in which to do so.

By screening for ACEs as early as possible, we can potentially prevent the physical, psychological, and economic cost of ACEs in children, which if left untreated will fuel another generation of high ACEs.

The Clinical and Child ACE Questionnaires

The ACE Clinical Questionnaire (Murphy, Dube, Steele, & Steele, 2007) was adapted from the ten categories of childhood adversity (Dube et al., 2003; Dube, Felitti, Croft, Edwards, & Giles, 2001) and developed for use in our clinical setting (A. Murphy, personal communication with S. Dube, 2007). We have established convergent validity between this questionnaire and the AAI (Murphy et al., 2014). As with the original ACE survey (Dube et al., 2001), questions about emotional and physical abuse, and household dysfunction were derived from the Conflict Tactics Scale (Straus, 1979); sexual abuse was determined based on four questions from Wyatt (1985); parental substance abuse was assessed with questions from Schoenborn (1991); and physical and emotional neglect variables were based on the Childhood Trauma Questionnaire (CTQ; Bernstein et al., 1994).

The Clinical ACE Questionnaire (Murphy et al., 2007) assesses the ten categories of adversity (Dube et al., 2002; Felitti et al., 1998). These include exposure to psychological, physical and sexual abuse, emotional and physical neglect, and what has been termed household dysfunction, specifically parental divorce or separation, untreated parental mental illness, parental alcohol or substance abuse, parental incarceration, and exposure to mother treated violently. An innovation in the Clinical ACE Questionnaire is the explicit reversal of the question regarding emotional neglect "During your first 18 years of life, there was no one who made you feel special, loved, or important," to instead ask "During your first 18 years of life, was there a parent who made you feel special, loved, or important?" Clinically, we believe this holds value as it opens up an avenue for identifying "angels in the nursery" who provided support that might buffer the effects of early adversity (Lieberman, Padrón, Van Horn, & Harris, 2005).

Building upon the original ACE study with an eye towards prevention, we developed the Child Clinical ACE Questionnaire (Murphy et al., 2007), with the same categories of questions, prefaced by, "Since your child was born, how often has he/she ... " This measure was created in an attempt to awaken in parents the idea that their children have the potential to have a different set of childhood experiences than they endured. This is particularly poignant for parents with high levels of ACEs. We have found that simply asking the parent the Clinical ACE Questionnaire and the Child Clinical ACE Questionnaire in succession has therapeutic value, as it can ignite the parent's capacity to reflect upon their children's current experiences in contrast to their own childhood experiences. A parent with an ACEs score of 7, learning that her child only has a 1, may be particularly motivated to engage with an integrated early childhood behavioral health specialist to prevent the intergenerational transmission and repetition of trauma.

Integrating Screening for Adverse Childhood Experiences in Primary Care Settings

As the inclusion of ACEs becomes part of trauma-informed screening, pediatricians, psychologists, social workers, and other mental health professionals often ask how to introduce questions about parent adverse childhood experiences within a pediatric primary care setting. Some providers have expressed fear that parents will be reluctant to consider why their own childhood has anything to do with their child's health, behavior, or development. Providers may express reluctance to query such private issues, because they question where to refer families should screening reveal high ACE scores.

Common Concerns with Asking About ACEs

The concerns we have heard expressed by providers regarding discussing ACEs with families can be divided into four themes. Comments include:

1. *Parents are coming in due to concerns about their child or just for a well-child visit. They do not expect to be asked about ACEs. They are a well-functioning middle class family.*

   In our experience of administering several hundred Clinical ACE and Child Clinical ACE Questionnaires (Murphy et al., 2007), parents rarely refuse to answer the questions, through we have had parents deny the presence of any ACEs. We suspect they are either dismissing their past experiences and/or are fearful that they will be reported to child protection agencies. It has been helpful to ask about ACEs particularly when there are concerns about behavior (i.e., ADHD, sleep problems, and speech delays). We remind providers that the original ACE study (Dube et al., 2003; Felitti et al., 1998) consisted of a middle class sample where close to 20 % of respondents reported more than four adverse childhood experiences, thus normalizing the prevalence and potential link between ACEs and behavioral concerns.

2. *I understand asking about parent ACEs, but what about child ACEs-aren't we mandated reporters?*

   By asking these questions we are creating an opportunity to better define and explain to parents that ACEs can make people physically and mentally ill. We have found it useful to instruct providers and parents on what constitutes abuse and neglect and how the components of household dysfunction are part of this body of research which has shown these behaviors to be harmful, contributing to physical and mental health problems throughout the life span.

3. *We can screen, but where do we send families when ACE scores are high?*

   The need for trauma-informed interventions cannot be overstated. There are several evidence-based interventions (Child Parent Psychotherapy; Lieberman, Ippen, & Van Horn, 2006; Attachment and Biobehavioral Catch-up; Bernard et al., 2012; Circle of Security, Hoffman; Marvin, Cooper, & Powell, 2006; Child First; Lowell, Carter, Godoy, Paulicin, & Briggs-Gowan, 2011) and evidence-informed treatment modalities (Group Attachment Based Intervention; GABI; Murphy et al., 2015), that specifically target parent–child relationship disturbances related to trauma. Perinatal and pediatric settings, indeed any health facility serving parents and children, should be familiar with the local opportunities for families to benefit from these evidence-informed and evidence-based treatments.

4. *Discussing findings from the ACE Questionnaire poses potential discomfort for providers.*

   We know that in the original ACE Study (Dube et al., 2003; Felitti et al., 1998), comprised of a community sample, close to 20 % of respondents reported more than four adverse childhood experiences, so we can surmise that for some clinicians the topic areas being discussed are particularly sensitive or even act as trauma triggers for them. Identifying one's own adverse childhood experiences may be a necessary step towards resolution so that they may provide support to patients. Education regarding the role of ACEs in mental and physical health should become prevalent in all trauma-informed behavioral healthcare training programs.

Summary and Recommendations

After two decades of findings from the ACE Study, the evidence is clear: early childhood adversity is common and contributes to negative health outcomes throughout the life span. After all we have learned from the ACE Study, our challenge now (as suggested by the AAP policy statement on toxic stress) is to find effective ways to prevent the intergenerational transmission of abuse, neglect, and dysfunction from occurring in the lives of future generations. While we realize that preventing ACEs cannot take a single pronged approach, our experiences as clinicians have helped us to understand what works and what does not work. Given our observations in assessing childhood adversity among high-risk families in a clinical setting, it was our intention to share all we have learned and explain the *how and why* of asking about ACEs, with an eye toward doing so in the pediatric setting. It is our hope that through this work, we can provide all practitioners a tool to better understand unresolved trauma in their patient population and make progress to end the intergenerational transmission of childhood adversity.

References

Academy of Pediatrics. (2012). Early childhood adversity, toxic stress, and the role of the pediatrician: Translating developmental science into lifelong health. *Pediatrics, 129*, 224–231.

Anda, R. F., Croft, J. B., Felitti, V. J., Nordenberg, D., Giles, W. H., Williamson, D. F., & Giovino, G. A. (1999). Adverse childhood experiences and smoking during adolescence and adulthood. *Journal of the American Medical Association, 282*(17), 1652–1658.

Belsky, J., & Fearon, R. P. (2002). Early attachment security, subsequent maternal sensitivity, and later child development: Does continuity in development depend upon continuity of caregiving? *Attachment & Human Development, 4*(3), 361–387.

Bernard, K., Dozier, M., Bick, J., Lewis-Morrarty, E., Lindhiem, O., & Carlson, E. (2012). Enhancing attachment organization among maltreated children: Results of a randomized clinical trial. *Child Development, 83*, 623–636.

Bernstein, D. P., Fink, L., Handelsman, L., Foote, J., Lovejoy, M., Wenzel, K., … Ruggiero, J. (1994). Initial reliability and validity of a new retrospective measure of child abuse and neglect. *The American Journal of Psychiatry, 151*(8), 1132–1136.

Berwick, D. M., Nolan, T. W., & Whittington, J. (2008). The triple aim: Care, health, and cost. *Health Affairs, 27*(3), 759–769.

Bowlby, J. (1969). *Attachment and loss* (Attachment, Vol. 1). New York, NY: Basic Books.

Bowlby, J. (1982). Attachment and loss: Retrospect and prospect. *American Journal of Orthopsychiatry, 52*(4), 664.

Bowlby, J. (1988). *A secure base: Parent-child attachment and healthy human development.* New York, NY: Basic Books.

Chapman, D. P., Whitfield, C. L., Felitti, V. J., Dube, S. R., Edwards, V. J., Robert, F., & Anda, R. F. (2004). Adverse childhood experiences and the risk of depressive disorders in adulthood. *Journal of Affective Disorders, 82*, 217–225.

De Bellis, M. D., Keshavan, M. S., Clark, D. B., Casey, B. J., Giedd, J. N., Boring, A. M., … Ryan, N. D. (1999). Developmental traumatology part II: Brain development. *Biological Psychiatry, 45*(10), 1271–1284.

Dube, S. R., Anda, R. F., Felitti, V. J., Chapman, D., Williamson, D. F., & Giles, W. H. (2001). Childhood abuse, household dysfunction and the risk of attempted suicide throughout the life span: Findings from Adverse Childhood Experiences Study. *Journal of the American Medical Association, 286*, 3089–3096.

Dube, S. R., Felitti, V. J., Croft, J. B., Edwards, V. J., & Giles, W. H. (2001). Growing up with parental alcohol abuse. *Child Abuse & Neglect, 25*, 1627–1640.

Dube, S. R., Anda, R. F., Felitti, V. J., Edwards, V. J., & Croft, J. B. (2002). Adverse childhood experiences and personal alcohol abuse as an adult. *Addictive Behaviors, 27*, 713–725.

Dube, S. R., Anda, R. F., Whitfield, C. L., Brown, D. W., Felitti, V. J., Dong, M., & Giles, W. H. (2005). Long-term consequences of childhood sexual abuse by gender of victim. *American Journal of Preventive Medicine, 28*(5), 430–438.

Dube, S., Cook, M., & Edwards, V. (2010). Peer reviewed: Health-related outcomes of adverse childhood experiences in Texas, 2002. *Preventing Chronic Disease, 7*(3).

Dube, S. R., Fairweather, D., Pearson, W. S., Felitti, V. J., Anda, R. F., & Croft, J. B. (2009). Cumulative childhood stress and autoimmune diseases in adults. *Psychosomatic Medicine, 71*(2), 243.

Dube, S. R., Felitti, V. J., Dong, M., Chapman, D. P., Giles, W., & Anda, R. F. (2003). Childhood abuse, neglect and household dysfunction and the risk of illicit drug use: The Adverse Childhood Experiences Study. *Pediatrics, 111*(3), 564–572.

Dube, S. R., Miller, J. W., Brown, D. W., Giles, W. H., Felitti, V. J., Dong, M., & Anda, R. F. (2006). Adverse childhood experiences and the association with ever using alcohol and initiating alcohol use during adolescence. *Journal of Adolescent Health, 38*(4), 444.e1–10.

Felitti V. J., Anda R. F., Nordenberg D., Williamson, D. F., Spitz, A. M., Edwards, V., & Marks, J. S. (1998). The relationship of adult health status to childhood abuse & household dysfunction. *American Journal of Preventive Medicine, 14*, 245–258

Groh, A. M., Fearon, R. P., Bakermans-Kranenburg, M. J., Van IJzendoorn, M. H., Steele, R. D., & Roisman, G. I. (2014). The significance of attachment security for children's social competence with peers: A meta-analytic study. *Attachment & Human Development, 16*(2), 103–136.

Hair, N., Hanson, J., Wolfe, B., & Pollak, S. (2015). Association of child poverty, brain development, and academic achievement. *JAMA Pediatrics, 169*(9), 822–829. doi:10.1001/jamapediatrics.2015.1475.

Harris, W. W., Putman, F. W., & Fairbank, J. A. (2004). *Mobilizing trauma resources for children.* Paper presented in part at the meeting of the Johnson and Johnson Pediatric Institute: Shaping the Future of Children's Health, San Juan, Puerto Rico, February 12–16, 2004.

Heckman, J. (2006). Skill formation and the economics of investing in disadvantaged children. *Science, 312*(5782), 1900–1902.

Hoffman, K. T., Marvin, R. S., Cooper, G., & Powell, B. (2006). Changing toddlers' and preschoolers' attachment classifications: The circle of security intervention. *Journal of Consulting and Clinical Psychology, 74*(6), 1017–1026. http://dx.doi.org/10.1037/0022-006X.74.6.1017.

Lehman, B. J., Taylor, S. E., Kiefe, C. I., & Seeman, T. E. (2009). Relationship of early life stress and psychological functioning to blood pressure in the CARDIA study. *Health Psychology, 28*(3), 338–346.

Lieberman, A. F., Ippen, C. G., & Van Horn, P. (2006). Child–parent psychotherapy: 6-month follow-up of a randomized controlled trial. *Journal of the American Academy of Child and Adolescent Psychiatry, 45*(8), 913–918.

Lieberman, A. F., Padrón, E., Van Horn, P., & Harris, W. W. (2005). Angels in the nursery: The intergenerational transmission of benevolent parental influences. *Infant Mental Health Journal, 26*(6), 504–520.

Lowell, D. I., Carter, A. S., Godoy, L., Paulicin, B., & Briggs-Gowan, M. J. (2011). A randomized controlled trial of child first: A comprehensive, home-based intervention translating research into early childhood practice. *Child Development, 82*(1), 193–208.

Lyons-Ruth, K., & Jacobvitz, D. (2008). Attachment disorganization: Genetic factors, parenting contexts, and developmental transformation from infancy to adulthood. In J. Cassidy & P. R.

Shaver (Eds.), *Handbook of attachment: Theory, research, and clinical applications* (2nd ed., pp. 666–697). New York, NY: Guilford Press.

Main, M., Goldwyn, R., & Hesse, E. (2003). *Adult attachment classification system version 7.2* (Unpublished manuscript). Berkeley, CA: University of California.

Main, M., Hesse, E., & Goldwyn, R. (2008). Studying differences in language use in recounting attachment history. In H. Steele & M. Steele (Eds.), *Clinical applications of the Adult Attachment Interview* (pp. 31–68). New York, NY: Guilford Press.

Main, M., Kaplan, N., & Cassidy, J. (1985). Security in infancy, childhood, and adulthood: A move to the level of representation. *Monographs of the Society for Research in Child Development, 50*, 66–104.

Meade, C. S., Kershaw, T. S., Hansen, N. B., & Sikkema, K. J. (2009). Long-term correlates of childhood abuse among adults with severe mental illness: Adult victimization, substance abuse, and HIV sexual risk behavior. *AIDS and Behavior, 13*(2), 207–216.

Murphy, A., Dube, S., Steele M., & Steele, H. (2007) *Clinical ACE and Child Clinical ACE Questionnaires* (Unpublished Manuscript).

Murphy, A., Steele, H., Bate, J., Nikitiades, A., Allman, B. Bonuck, K., … Steele, M. (2015). Group Attachment Based Intervention: Trauma Informed Care for Families with Adverse Childhood Experiences. *Family and Community Health, 38*(3), 268–279.

Murphy, A., Steele, M., Dube, S. R., Bate, J., Bonuck, K., Meissner, P., … Steele, H. (2014). Adverse childhood experiences (ACEs) questionnaire and adult attachment interview (AAI): Implications for parent child relationships. *Child Abuse & Neglect, 38*(2), 224–233.

Pederson, D. R., Gleason, K. E., Moran, G., & Bento, S. (1998). Maternal attachment representations, maternal sensitivity, and the infant–mother attachment relationship. *Developmental Psychology, 34*(5), 925.

Schoenborn, C. A. (1991). Exposure to alcoholism in the family: United States, 1988. *Advance Data from Vital and Health Statistics, 30*(205), 1–13.

Slade, A. (2005). Parental reflective functioning: An introduction. *Attachment & Human Development, 7*(3), 269–281.

Steele, H., Bate, J., Steele, M., Dube, S. R., Danskin, K., Knafo, H., … Murphy, A. (2016). Adverse childhood experiences, poverty and parenting stress. *Canadian Journal of Behavioral Science, 48*(1), 32–38.

Steele, H., Steele, M., & Fonagy, P. (1996). Associations among attachment classification of mothers, fathers and their infants. *Child Development, 67*, 541–555.

Stein, M. B., Koverola, C., Hanna, C., Torchia, M. G., & McClarty, B. (1997). Hippocampal volume in women victimized by childhood sexual abuse. *Psychological Medicine, 27*(4), 951–959.

Straus, M. A. (1979). Measuring intrafamily conflict and violence: The conflict tactics (CT) scales. *Journal of Marriage and the Family, 41*(1), 75–88.

Teicher, M. H., Ito, Y., Glod, C. A., Andersen, S. L., Dumont, N., & Ackerman, E. (1997). Preliminary evidence for abnormal cortical development in physically and sexually abused children using EEG coherence and MRI. *Annals of the New York Academy of Sciences, 821*(1), 160–175.

Van der Kolk, B. A. (1994). The body keeps the score: Memory and the evolving psychobiology of posttraumatic stress. *Harvard Review of Psychiatry, 1*(5), 253–265.

van IJzendoorn, M. H. (1995). Adult attachment representations, parental responsiveness, and infant attachment: A meta-analysis on the predictive validity of the Adult Attachment Interview. *Psychological Bulletin, 117*, 387–403.

Ward, M. J., & Carlson, E. A. (1995). Associations among adult attachment representations, maternal sensitivity, and infant mother attachment in a sample of adolescent mothers. *Child Development, 66*(1), 69–79.

Wyatt, G. E. (1985). The sexual abuse of Afro-American and white-American women in childhood. *Child Abuse & Neglect, 9*(4), 507–519.

Chapter 3
The Economics of Child Development

Andrew D. Racine

Abstract In recent years our understanding of the science of child development has increased in sophistication from the standpoint of neuroscience, cognition, psychology, and molecular biology. In conjunction with these advances, the discipline of economics has contributed its own important insights with salient policy implications. This chapter reviews the underlying theory motivating the recent economic literature regarding the importance of early investments in child development. In particular, it characterizes the application of human capital theory to the arena of early childhood skill development. It highlights some of the methodological challenges facing economic evaluations of early child development interventions and summarizes the empirical findings derived from both highly controlled model programs as well as larger scale "real-world" interventions designed to augment child cognitive and social emotional skills. The conclusion is that from an economic standpoint, the returns to investment in early child development are substantial and compare favorably to alternative uses of equivalent resources.

Keywords Human capital • Child development • Cost-benefit analysis • Economic evaluation

Introduction

The science of child development has experienced a profound transformation in recent years as a result of insights gleaned from disciplines as diverse as developmental psychology, imaging science, epigenetics, molecular biology, epidemiology, and pediatrics (Shonkoff & Phillips, 2000). Scholars from diverse backgrounds are formulating a nuanced and sophisticated vision of how genes and the environment interact to produce the neuroanatomic and physiological templates from which cognitive, behavioral, and social-emotional outcomes in children emerge (Davidson & McEwen, 2012). As researchers illuminate the importance of preconception, fetal, neonatal, and early

A.D. Racine, M.D., Ph.D. (✉)
Montefiore Medicine, Bronx, NY, USA
e-mail: aracine@montefiore.org

© Springer International Publishing Switzerland 2016   17
R.D. Briggs (ed.), *Integrated Early Childhood Behavioral Health
in Primary Care*, DOI 10.1007/978-3-319-31815-8_3

childhood influences on lifelong developmental trajectories, new areas of inquiry present themselves to clinical and social scientists who help translate these findings into practical real-world applications.

Economics is an area of scientific inquiry that offers its own pertinent contributions to this evolving portrait. Traditionally, and in its most narrow sense, economic analysis sets out to answer the question of how individuals or firms should allocate scarce resources efficiently to maximize either utility or profit (Mankiw, 2007). Through theoretical modeling and empirical research, economists help policy makers appreciate the implications of allocative decisions on a variety of choices such as the use of public funds for health, infrastructure or defense purposes or the enactment of tax policies that encourage socially desirable outcomes such as energy conservation or smoking cessation. Given the traditional role played by economics, what insights can we derive from this discipline that will add to our understanding of child development and inform our conceptual models as well as our approach to policy interventions? To help answer these questions, this chapter will review both the theory and the application of economic analysis as it pertains to our understanding of the trajectory of child development, and the provision of early childhood services.

The chapter will be divided into four sections. We begin with an outline of the theoretical construct that underlies an economic approach to child development as it has evolved within the framework of human capital theory. Next we outline ways in which the methodological approach of economists helps us evaluate the empirical literature. With this background we can then turn our attention to cost-benefit studies on the impact of specific child development programs. Finally we will suggest some of the policy implications that these economic insights point to and offer some concluding remarks.

The Economic Theory of Early Child Development

The most valuable of all capital is that invested in human beings; and of that capital the most precious part is the result of the care and influence of the mother...

Alfred Marshall *Principles of Economics* (VI, IV, 11)

Marshall wrote those words in 1890, though the antecedents of what has come to be known as human capital theory reach as far back as Adam Smith who wrote in *The Wealth of Nations* about, "...the acquired and useful abilities of all inhabitants or members of the society....which is a capital fixed and realized as it were in his person." The latter day revisitation of these ideas owes much to the work of Gary Becker with his publication of *Human Capital* in 1975. Becker's seminal insight was that individuals in a market economy, far from being simply consumers of goods and services, were themselves producers. They combine commodity purchases with their own time and environmental inputs to produce satisfaction for themselves. Part of the time they spend toward this goal of increased satisfaction can be thought of as *investment time* during which they improve their own ability to be more productive, notably through education (Becker, 1975). This self-improvement investment activity augments a stock of capabilities referred to as human capital—stored intangible wealth that will generate an ongoing stream of benefits to the individual over time.

At its essence human capital theory reimagines individuals as firms engaged in the production of their own capabilities. Like firms, they combine a set of inputs in different combinations to secure a specific outcome, namely an improved future state either of health, income, or general satisfaction. Also like firms, individuals must balance their available resources in pursuit of optimal production outcomes. Sometimes to afford the inputs they desire they may even have to borrow in the present against returns that will come about at some future date. In this view individuals make decisions based on tastes, innate endowment, time preferences, and disposable income that enable them to augment their cognitive, social, and physical health in such a way as to earn future returns on those investments.

A classic example of this behavior involves decisions to invest in education. Individuals choose to pursue higher education because that investment results in the likelihood of greater future earnings. They pay or even borrow money in the present for tuition with the expectation that those payments will afford them a higher future stream of income than what they might have achieved without that educational investment. Beyond formal education, one can also augment one's human capital through on the job training; through investments in health like better nutrition, exercise, and avoiding risky behaviors; through migration to geographic locales with better economic prospects, etc.

From the standpoint of child development it was important for human capital theorists to frame the question from the child's point of view (Leibowitz, 1974). Taking a child centric approach required incorporation of a time dimension for investment decisions and a broad sense of where such investments might originate. Building on earlier work (Becker and Tomes, 1986; Ben Porath, 1967), recent authors recognized that the development of children's capacities involved a series of different inputs from various sources: genetic endowment, parents, other adults, child care institutions, nutrition, books, etc. applied sequentially over time to generate both cognitive and noncognitive capacities that would govern a child's behavior and eventual adult health status. The best known proponent of this application of human capital theory to child development is Nobel Prize winning economist James Heckman who developed an economic model that set out to explain human capital development in children over time.

Heckman's model contains several salient features that conform elegantly to empirical observations generated in the clinical literature. These features have been recently summarized (Conti & Heckman, 2012) and include three basic elements. First, the outcome of child well-being in a given period involves a vector of capabilities that is multidimensional but primarily focuses on cognitive abilities, noncognitive personality traits (temperament, attentiveness, perseverance, impulse control, sociability, etc.), health capacities, and effort. One important implication of this aspect of the model is that various combinations of these inputs can result in similar outcomes so that even programs that have no discernible impact on IQ result in substantive improvement in child outcomes through the impact they have on noncognitive characteristics.

The second feature of the model is that it is dynamic over time so that the outcome for a child in period T is a function of that child's capacities as they existed in the previous time period plus investments, environmental inputs, and parental traits. Several implications derive from this aspect of the model. First, other things being equal, higher levels of capacity in one time period beget higher levels in the subsequent period. Skills beget skills in a process that the authors refer to as "self-productivity." Healthier children with a higher stock of human capital, for instance, can benefit more from educational investments than unhealthy children (Cunha & Heckman, 2007).

A third implication of the model is that because investments take place in different time periods, the effectiveness of investments in child human capital formation may vary over time. It is conceivable, indeed likely, that this effectiveness is not constant and that the same level of investment in one period may be disproportionally effective when compared to the impact it might have in other periods. These periods when human capital investments are particularly effective are referred to as "sensitive" periods. At the extreme there may even be some periods where investments *must* occur if they are to have any positive impact on the outcome whatsoever. For example, young children with untreated amblyopia, a condition that impedes an eye's ability to focus, may permanently lose the ability to see through the affected eye regardless of how much investment is put toward attempting to correct this in later periods. Just as there are sensitive periods during which investment in child human capital has large potential rewards, the converse is also true. Parental inputs into the skill formation of children may become less effective in later years than they are during infancy and toddlerhood (Heckman & Masterov, 2007).

A fourth intriguing aspect of the model of human capital formation in children is that not only do investments complement already developed capacities, meaning that children with higher levels of skills benefit more from the same level of investment than do children with less skill development, but investments in one time period influence the effectiveness of investments that occur in later periods since they enhance the level of skills to which the subsequent investments are applied. In this regard early investments make later investments more effective. This "dynamic complementarity" of investment activities has important policy implications much as compound interest does where early investments compound over time to yield greater returns than would occur if the exact same level of investment were to be delayed to a later period (Heckman, 2007).

Taken as a whole, the human capital model of skill formation in children would lead to certain predictions regarding how development should manifest itself in the real world. One would expect the results from empirical studies to show that stocks of human capital or capabilities matter. The higher the stock in terms of cognitive, noncognitive, health, and genetic endowment, the more successful would be the expected developmental trajectory over time. It should also become evident that the earlier that investments are made in human capital formation for children, the greater the eventual return. This doesn't mean that it would prove impossible to augment stocks of human capital in later time periods but it may be more expensive to do so, and the returns on this investment may be much less than if the same intensity of investment is applied earlier in development. Investments can be directed to improve noncognitive as well as cognitive skill sets and thereby result in equivalent boosts in outcome. Finally, the model would predict that, while the birth lottery is important, initial endowments are not destiny. Genetic and parental initial conditions are highly alterable depending upon the level of investment that takes place at critical junctures and that is ongoing particularly early in a child's lifetime.

To see how predictive propositions are or are not borne out by the empirical literature it is first necessary to appreciate that robust economic analysis requires certain methodological attributes in order to discern whether or not a given set of data are meaningfully interpretable. It is to these methodological considerations that we may briefly turn our attention before embarking on a review of the cost-benefit studies that have been conducted on real-world programs devoted to child development.

Methods

When considering what is known about the biology and physiology of early childhood development, one overwhelming real-world question that arises is: can we do anything to influence the trajectory of these developmental outcomes and if so what? In this regard, economists have something unique to offer. Their preferred approach reduces the outcome analysis to a very specific question. They ask not whether a given intervention improves a specific developmental outcome or not but rather do the gains from that intervention exceed the resources expended to execute it?

To answer that question economists have elaborated analytic tools that evaluate costs of interventions and compare them to outcomes measured in several ways (Petitti, 2000). In *cost minimization* studies different interventions that achieve the exact same result are compared to one another to see which one can be performed at the least expense. In a related approach, *cost-effectiveness* analyses allow the outcomes to vary between different interventions but pose the question which program achieves results at the lowest cost per unit of outcome produced. A third analytic approach and one that will be explored in more detail in this section is the *cost-benefit* analysis. Economists generally apply cost-benefit analysis when the costs, in dollar terms, to conduct an intervention are compared to the benefits, also expressed in dollars, derived from the intervention. This balance of costs and benefits is then presented either as a net amount, indicating that the benefits either do or do not exceed the costs of the intervention, as a ratio of benefits to costs, or as a rate of return on the intervention over time (Levin & McEwan, 2001). While some use this methodology to refer to specific programs as "cost-beneficial" meaning that the net benefits of a program are more than zero, the true application of the technique resides in using it to compare different programs to one another. For an economist, the relevant question is, "If I have a dollar to spend on improving child development, am I better off spending it on this program or that one?" Where, in other words, do I achieve the highest return per dollar invested? If I don't choose wisely, my ultimate decisions result in an inefficient use of resources and I am, by definition, foregoing a superior state of the world that would result from a different set of decisions.

On the face of it, this type of analysis is quite appealing but it is a challenging construct to apply rigorously (Gold, Siegel, et al. 1996). There are a series of important challenges to conducting or evaluating a cost-benefit analysis. The first and perhaps most important is deciding which programs should be studied. To understand the marginal impact of a specific program or intervention it is imperative that a group comparable to those involved in the program but who are not exposed to the intervention also be part of the analysis. In this way, the impact of the program itself can be isolated and measured. In ideal circumstances, to achieve a robust comparison group, random assignment of participants from among a studied population should be part of the design. This cannot always be the case and when it is not analysts must be wary of the possibility that those individuals who chose to participate in the program being analyzed are systematically different from those in the control group who did not participate. Self-selection in non-randomized designs can introduce bias that will compromise a cost-benefit analysis by making it difficult to ascertain exactly what observed benefits are due to the program and what benefits are due to unobserved but critical attributes of those who chose to participate in the program compared to those who declined. See more in Chap. 10 of this volume, focused on evaluation methods.

A second vital criterion of any cost-benefit analysis is determining from whose perspective the analysis should be performed (Torrance, Siegel, & Luce, 1996). One can consider the private costs and benefits to the participant of enrolling in an early child development program; one might focus on the governmental outlays for such an endeavor; or, as is often done, one takes into account all the public as well as private costs and benefits and adopts a societal perspective for the analysis.

A third important challenge is finding a way to monetize all potential costs and benefits of a particular program (Gold, Patrick, et al. 1996). Usually the costs are not difficult to enumerate and associate with specific dollar amounts but monetizing the benefits may be much more problematic. What is the value of an extra five IQ points in dollars? How much are improvements in noncognitive skills like attentiveness worth? The approach taken in most evaluations is to focus on the tangible impact of these developmental achievements with regard to graduation rates from high school, grade retention frequency, college attendance, etc. Because the dollar costs and benefits of these outcomes are more tractable, it is possible to enumerate them and compare them to the program costs directly.

The fourth consideration for conducting cost-benefit analyses is to ensure that all possible benefits are accounted for and that often means, with respect to programs for child development, making sure that the follow-up time is sufficient to capture the downstream impacts of the investments and that attrition of subjects from the analysis is minimized to the extent possible. Some cost-benefit analyses, for example, include the impact of early childhood programs on the likelihood of subsequent involvement in the criminal justice system. Others consider future tax payments of children once they become adults. These are decisions that have profound implications for whether or not a given program may or may not result in net positive returns. Because benefits are future events, the length of follow-up and the magnitude of attrition of the original cohort of subjects represent significant threats to the validity of any study of child development.

Fifth, because benefits accrue in the future but costs are dispensed in the present, there must be a method used to discount the future benefits in order to be able to compare them directly to the present day costs. The choice of discount rate will have important ramifications since steeper discount rates make future benefits less valuable relative to current expenditures than do more modest discount rates. Related to this point is the manner in which the results of the cost-benefit analysis are expressed. Asking simply whether the program, "pays for itself" will not take into account the rapidity with which the net result is achieved. By contrast, the internal rate of return calculation (IRR) will do this. If the results from one program become manifest earlier than the results from a separate program with equivalent benefits, the IRR will be higher for the first program despite this equivalency.

Sixth, since the quality of the inputs to an intervention has significant implications for the outcomes generated by that intervention, measuring and quantifying that quality is an important methodological challenge. Some quality features are easier to quantify than others so that elements such as staff to child ratios or the educational qualifications of providers in a specific program can be captured with little difficulty. Other quality features such as the educational approach adopted by a program or the training inputs for those interacting with the children tend to be less tangible.

Finally, all assumptions for a specific cost-benefit analysis have a degree of uncertainty associated with them and by relaxing the assumptions for a specific analysis the impact of those assumptions on the outcomes achieved can be tested directly.

Given the number of different elements associated with any given cost-benefit analysis, it is not surprising that comparing one of them to another can be fraught with complications. There are authors who have attempted to summarize series of cost-benefit analyses to arrive at summative judgments about the effectiveness of early childhood development interventions, but economists have been alert to some of the methodological complexities associated with attempting to aggregate the results of various studies.

Some analyses, as we shall see below, are conducted on randomized controlled trials with small sample sizes. Others evaluate large interventions conducted in less controlled environments with different subject characteristics and different follow-up periods. They may include different sets of benefits in their analyses. Since different studies can sometimes come to different conclusions about the effectiveness of a given intervention, it is important to recognize what portion of those different findings results from differences in methods as opposed to differences in what is being measured, namely the effectiveness of the intervention. When the methods used to evaluate a program are correlated with the results of the evaluation, there is a danger of confusing the effects of the program with effects of how the program evaluation was conducted. If, for example, a well-conducted randomized controlled trial had long-term follow-ups that incorporated a large array of possible outcomes including criminal justice outcomes whereas a larger observational study conducted under real-world conditions did not include the same number of benefits or did not follow subjects as long or had greater attrition over time, it might be concluded that the type, quality, or intensity of the intervention studied was the reason for the different outcomes rather than the methods used to evaluate the different programs. These confounding moderators have been well articulated in recent years (Lipsey, 2003) and bear thinking about as we review what is known about the empirical literature on early childhood interventions in the next section.

Empirical Findings

> ...*a growing body of program evaluations shows that early childhood programs have the potential to generate government savings that more than repay their costs and produce returns to society as a whole that outpace most public and private investments.*
>
> Kilburn and Kroly—The Economics of Early Childhood Policy

Economists, like other social scientists, have a particular respect for the randomized controlled trial design. Considered the methodological gold standard (see Chap. 10 in this volume for more detail), it is no surprise that many of the most rigorous cost-benefit analyses published to date are studies examining the few randomized controlled trials of early childhood interventions. Economic evaluations of the best known early child intervention studies generally reach similar conclusions that the economic returns on these programs are substantial and the longer the time course over which benefits are examined, the larger the return (Barnett, 2011).

Among the best known interventions to have been subject to rigorous evaluations, the HighScope Perry Preschool Program, the Carolina Abecedarian Project, the Chicago Child-Parent Center program (Reynolds, 2000), the Nurse-Family Partnership program (Aos, Lieb, Mayfield, Miller, & Pennucci, 2004), Head Start (Puma, Bell, Cook, & Heid, 2010), Healthy Steps (Zuckerman, Parker, Kaplan-Sanoff, Augustyn, & Barth, 2004), and several international interventions (Engle et al., 2011; Gertler et al., 2013) bear scrutiny. The first two because of the rigorous randomized controlled trial design of the interventions and the others due to the "real-world" activity they represent.

Begun in the early 1960s at the Perry Elementary School in Ypsilanti Michigan, the Perry Preschool Program randomized 123 low-income African-American 3-year-old preschoolers with IQ scores below 85 into five cohorts for a study that lasted 2 years (Schweinhart, Barnes, & Weikart, 1993). The 58 children in the intervention group received a 2.5 h preschool program 5 days a week for 30 weeks of the school year and weekly 90 min home visits by teachers to encourage parents to interact with their children, while the control group of 65 children enrolled in regular kindergarten at the Perry Elementary School at age 5. All of the teachers in the project were licensed public school teachers with baccalaureate degrees in education and training in early childhood education and the teacher/student ratio was 1:6. In follow-up studies, the participants have been assessed up to the age of 40 when they provided detailed information regarding schooling, economic activities, incarceration experiences, and welfare program participation.

The Perry Preschool Program has been subject to several cost-benefit analyses (Barnett, 1985a, 1985b, 1993; Belfield, Nores, Barnett, & Schweinhart, 2006; Nores, Belfield, Barnett, & Schweinhart, 2005; Rolnick & Grunewald, 2003) that estimated the rate of return to participation in the program to be between 2 and 16 % depending upon the length of follow-up. In 2010, James Heckman and colleagues conducted the most rigorous economic evaluation of the program that took into account several shortcomings of previous analyses. In particular there were threats to the validity of findings from the initial cost benefit studies based on violations of the randomization protocol in the original study, the fact that some data were missing for follow-up assessments, the absence of standard errors to characterize the confidence intervals around cost and benefit findings, the lack of accounting for the cost of taxation to finance the intervention program, and that when monetizing the benefits of crime avoidance, educational advancement, and welfare participation earlier studies relied on national as opposed to local cost data. Heckman's reanalysis corrected for these shortcomings and found the rate of return on the Perry Preschool Program to be in the range of 7–10 %. Stated another way, this reinterpretation would suggest that, using a 3 % discount rate, every dollar invested in the Perry Preschool Program results in a present value return to society of between $7 and $12 (Heckman, Moon, Pinto, Savelyev, & Yavitz, 2010).

The second randomized controlled trial that has been extensively evaluated from a cost-benefit standpoint is the Carolina Abecedarian Project (Campbell, Helms, Sparling, & Ramey, 1998). In this early child development intervention begun in the late 1970s, 112 African-American children mostly at risk for cognitive and social/emotional delay were randomized at 6 weeks of age into either an intervention or a control group. Both groups received nutritional and medical support but the intervention group also enrolled in a center-based preschool program that operated full day schedules 5 days per week for 50 weeks per year from enrollment through to kindergarten entry. The curriculum, delivered to these infants and children with 3:1 child to staff ratios for infants and 6:1 ratios for preschoolers, was specifically attentive to developmental advancement (Sparling & Lewis, 1979, 1984). There was no home visitation element in this program in contrast to the Perry Preschool Program and the follow-up evaluations assessed participants up through age 21.

Cost-benefit evaluation of the Abecedarian Project enumerated benefits that included earnings of participants and their progeny, maternal earnings, savings in elementary and secondary school from avoidance of special education outlays, health benefits from reduced smoking, and lessened participation in public assistance programs (Barnett & Masse, 2007). The evaluation did not find differences between participants and nonparticipants related to crime outcomes and so did not include this in the cost-benefit calculation, nor did the evaluation count the benefits of the child care services provided by the program as benefits to the participants. Taken together the net rate of return for the Abecedarian project participants was, nevertheless, calculated conservatively at above 7 % putting this estimate remarkably close to the one calculated for the Perry Preschool Program despite the differences in the length, intensity, and content of the two interventions.

One of the critiques of the cost-benefit evaluations conducted on these randomized controlled trials was that the real world does not act like a randomized controlled trial and whether or not the effectiveness of early childhood interventions as applied in a real-world setting would generate equivalent savings remained an open question. An important example of this cautionary posture is exemplified in a randomized controlled trial of Head Start conducted by the US Government from 2002 to 2006 that followed 5000 3- and 4-year olds from 84 Head Start grantee/delegate agencies who were randomly assigned either to receive Head Start services or not to receive them. While a set of intermediary outcomes indicated favorable experiences for those who received Head Start services, there were few differences between the two groups that were discernable after the first grade with respect to cognitive or noncognitive skills (Puma et al., 2010).

Although this Head Start evaluation had the virtue of evaluating a real-world application in a randomized design, a notable shortcoming of the analysis was that the follow-up period was very short so that many of the benefits identified in the earlier two randomized controlled trials could not be ascertained. For this reason, studies that examined the Chicago Child-Parent Center Program (CPC) were of considerable interest to the social science and policy communities. For unlike the HighScope Perry Preschool Program or the Carolina Abecedarian Project, the CPC was a federally funded multisite intervention that operated at 24 sites in the Chicago public school system. Unlike the Head Start Impact study, these participants have been followed up for many years. In a quasi-experimental design the program enrolled its first cohort of 989 3 and 4 year old low-income children born in 1980 and followed them over time together with 550 children from the same neighborhoods matched on age and socioeconomic status who were enrolled in full day kindergarten in randomly selected schools associated with the Child-Parent Centers. Some of the comparison children were enrolled in Head Start and others were in home care.

Children enrolled in the CPC received instruction centered on the acquisition of basic language and math skills delivered by licensed Chicago public school teachers with at least a bachelor's degree in 3-h sessions 5 days a week during the 9 month school year with a 6 week summer session in addition. Services continued in two thirds of the sites for children in the 1st and 2nd grades and through 3rd grade in the remainder of the sites. The child to staff ratios were 17:2 for the preschool program and all instructors were certified in early childhood education. An important component of the program was an intensive element of parental involvement in the school context with the participants and the teachers. An outreach program was also included as were health and nutrition services for participants.

Several cost-benefit analyses of the program have been conducted at the point where the children had reached their 21st birthdays (Lee, Aos, & Miller, 2008; Reynolds, Temple, Robertson, & Mann, 2002; Temple & Reynolds, 2007) and one which calculated net benefits through to age 27 (Reynolds, Temple, White, Ou, & Robertson, 2011). In the most recent study the authors calculated the net present value of the program taking into account five categories of benefits including savings related to reduced expenditures on special education, decreased juvenile and adult criminal justice expenditures, reductions in expenditures associated with child welfare system payments, averted expenditures for victims of crimes due to lower rates of arrests, and increased projected future earnings and tax collections resulting from higher rates of high school completion. The analysis was careful to distinguish benefits that accrued primarily to the participants, those that were enjoyed by the general public as a result of the actions of the participants, and benefits to society at large consisting of the sum of the two former categories. The study found in follow-up that participants exceeded comparison group children with respect to their school achievement and high school graduation rates, avoidance of remedial educational services and involvement with the criminal justice system, and had fewer reports of child maltreatment or neglect.

Total present value costs of the preschool program were calculated at $8512 per participant. Total society benefits as a result of participation in the program included $5317 savings in special education, $24,240 in juvenile crime victim costs averted, $28,844 increased earnings, $18,222 adult crime victim costs saved, and other savings for a total social return of $92,220. Subtracting the program costs yielded a net benefit to society of $83,708. Stated another way, every dollar invested in the CPC preschool program resulted in a net return to society of $17.88 for boys and $2.67 for girls, the difference being largely due to comparative rates of involvement with the criminal justice system between males and females. In a sensitivity analysis the authors found that, unsurprisingly, these findings were sensitive to the assumed discount rate, that is the rate which future costs and benefits are discounted relative to present costs. Even at rates as high as 7 % the preschool program returned net benefits to society. The discount rate at which benefits to society exactly equaled costs (or the IRR of the program) was calculated to be 18 %.

In summarizing the findings of cost-benefit analyses conducted on the most rigorously designed early childhood intervention programs where participants have been followed for substantial periods of time, the benefits derived from participation in these programs significantly exceed the costs to deliver the services. Rates of return from an economic perspective to society as a whole compare very favorably with alternative uses for the resources devoted to these activities (Dalziel, Halliday & Segal, 2015).

Direct human capital investments in early childhood education as described above are not the only avenues that have been explored to advance the developmental capacities of young children. Home visiting and integration of developmental and social emotional services in the context of primary care pediatrics are two other notable modalities that have been subject to some economic evaluation. One of the best-known home visiting intervention programs that has been extensively studied is the Nurse-Family Partnership program (NFP) developed by David Olds originally in Elmira, New York and later replicated in Memphis, Tennessee and Denver, Colorado. From the first of these programs launched in the late 1970s with a sample of 400 low-income Whites through the late 1980s with a sample of 1178 predominantly African-Americans in Tennessee to the 735 largely Latino participants in the Colorado version, the program maintained remarkable fidelity to its initial purpose: to promote better pregnancy outcomes through improved prenatal health of mothers; to improve children's health and development through partnering with parents; and to maximize parents' economic self-sufficiency. Focusing on low-income women and their first babies, the program involved nurse home visitations every 2 weeks beginning at 25 weeks gestation and continuing with decreasing frequency until the infants were 18–24 months of age at which point the visits were approximately every 6 weeks (Olds, Henderson, Tatelbaum, & Chamberlin, 1986). In a randomized controlled design for the Elmira sample compared to control individuals, those assigned to the most comprehensive visit schedule

were found to have made better use of community support services, to be more consci-
entious in attending prenatal classes, to report better family and partner relationships,
and to report fewer personal problems. Young adolescents delivered babies with higher
birth weights and smokers who were assigned to nurse visitations had fewer preterm
deliveries. In longer term follow-up (Haskins & Barnett, 2010; Olds et al. 1997) those
who had experienced nurse visits made less frequent use of public assistance programs
in the Elmira and Memphis trials and had higher maternal earnings in all three initial
study cities than those who were not visited.

No comprehensive cost-benefit calculations were attempted in the initial evaluations of the NFP outcomes but in 2003 the Washington State Legislature asked the
Washington State Institute for Public Policy (www.wsipp.wa.gov) to evaluate a series
of child intervention strategies to see which ones had beneficial effects on education
outcomes of participants, substance abuse, criminal outcomes, child abuse and neglect
rates and teen pregnancy outcomes. Their review of the literature on NFP outcomes
coupled with a detailed monetization algorithm calculated that present value average
costs of participation in the program equaled $9118 whereas the net present value of
benefits equaled $26,298 for a net return of $2.88 for every dollar invested (Aos et al.,
2004). It should be noted that these cost-benefit calculations were based on outcome
data largely generated by evaluations conducted by the NFP program's originators. As
the Nurse Family Partnership model matures beyond the demonstration sites to a
broader diffusion throughout the country (it is currently being applied in over 43 states
in the USA, see http://www.nursefamilypartnership.org/about/program-history) continued economic evaluations of the program will be important.

A major theme that runs through most of the human capital development literature is the importance of beginning investments as early as possible. This is one of
the guiding principles of having NFP visits begin before delivery. A second approach
that also recognizes the value of very early capacity building is a program called
Healthy Steps that was developed in the 1990s through a collaboration between
Boston University and the Commonwealth Fund (Minkovitz et al., 2003). Using
specialists trained in parenting support and early child development working collaboratively with pediatricians, the Healthy Steps model uses scheduled well child
visits during the first 3 years of life to augment the services offered in the pediatrics
office. The goal of the program is to enhance parenting skills, build on identified
strengths of caregiver infant dyads, inject awareness of infant and child development into the anticipatory guidance offered by practicing clinicians, and address
potential risk factors such as maternal stress and depression as early as possible.
Using a combination of home visits, scheduled interactions with the Healthy Steps
specialist in the medical practice, an advice telephone service, and group parenting
sessions, the program represents a collaborative human capital investment model
centered in primary care pediatric offices.

In 2009, Piotrowski et al. conducted a meta-analysis of 13 published Healthy
Steps evaluations. There were 15 sites across the USA where HS programs were
examined, and six of those sites included a randomized controlled design. Despite
the relatively modest $900 per participant per year cost of HS programs and some
evidence of improved parenting practices in discipline, play activities, sleep

positioning, and reading, there have been no rigorous cost-benefit follow-up studies of this intervention model to date. It remains to be seen, therefore, how HS compares in net benefits to the other modalities reviewed previously.

The question of how generalizable findings from programs conducted in the USA are to international contexts is one not to be neglected. Compared with the economic benefits estimated from the first three programs reviewed in this section, international evaluations reveal equivalent economic benefits to early childhood investment in developing countries (Burger, 2010; Gertler et al., 2013). Engle et al. (2011) conducted a meta-analysis of 15 studies that looked at parenting interventions ranging from home visits, group sessions with parents, primary care visit interventions, or combinations of these modalities. They found that preschool enrollment substantially decreased the schooling attainment gap for participants and when monetizing the impact of this educational gain alone without taking other benefits into account, the authors calculated that benefit: cost ratios (returns to these interventions), depending upon the assumed discount rate, ranged from 6.4 to 17.6.

While we have reviewed only a small sampling of the hundreds of early child intervention programs that have had some degree of economic evaluation in the past several years, the preponderance of evidence that has been amassed in two decades of analysis strongly signals that when the benefits to society are comprehensively catalogued and properly discounted, the net benefits of these investments in early childhood development compared very favorably with potential alternative uses. This is the question that economists set for themselves: given a marginal dollar to invest, where does it make sense from an efficiency standpoint to target that dollar. Early childhood development programs—whether delivered in a highly controlled model program, incorporated into large-scale interventions in existing structures, situated as stand-alone educational interventions, fashioned into home visiting structures, or integrated into primary care pediatrics—from all available evidence represent powerful claims on scarce resources from an economic efficiency standpoint.

Policy Implications and Conclusions

> *The conventional view of economic development typically includes company headquarters, office towers, entertainment centers, and professional sports stadiums and arenas...in the future any proposed economic development list should have early childhood development at the top.*
>
> Rolnick and Grunewald—Early Childhood Development: Economic
> Development with a High Public Return

Given what has been reviewed regarding the economic returns on investment in young children, the obvious policy question that arises is: if this is such a good investment, why is it not occurring already? In rational markets, capital investments follow potential returns until such time as the return on a dollar invested in one activity is no greater than it would be if invested in an alternative. This notion that a well-functioning market will efficiently distribute available capital to equalize investment returns is predicated on the fact that the market in question is indeed "well-functioning." In economic terms, "well-functioning" has a particular meaning in that specific conditions must exist in order for a market to work efficiently. Among other things, there should be few if any liquidity constraints on the availability of capital so that interested individuals or firms should be able to access investment opportunities by borrowing if necessary to actualize their investments. Additionally the information available to the various actors in the market must be such that purchasers and sellers have access to the same data. If information asymmetries exist, price signals, among other things, do not operate efficiently. Finally, there should be few if any externalities in the market meaning that one's decision to purchase a good or a service should not have either significant positive or negative effects on those not party to the transaction. If my decision to purchase and smoke cigarettes induces a loss of welfare to the people around me that I am not responsible to pay for, then the full social cost of my purchase is not reflected in the price I am paying and I am quite likely to purchase more cigarettes than I might otherwise do if I were subject to the full cost of my actions. Conversely, the positive externalities associated with vaccinations result in fewer vaccines being purchased than would be the case if the full social benefits of vaccination (including the benefits to those who might come into contact with the individual who has been vaccinated) were taken into account.

The existence of each of these market failures in the context of investments in early childhood development initiatives is well known. The credit constraint that children face in their developmental pathway is not an inability to borrow in order to finance tuition for college. It is rather, in the words of James Heckman, "…the inability of children to borrow against future income to buy a parental environment that will allow them to fulfill their potential. It is the accident of birth." (Heckman & Masterov, 2007). It is also the case that access to reliable information regarding the quality of preschool programs is tenuous for most parents such that their ability to choose rationally among competing alternatives is compromised (Currie, 2001). Finally, the positive externalities of investing in the cognitive and social emotional development of children in the form of crime avoided (Yoshikawa, 1995), higher tax revenues (Heckman et al., 2010), and improved adult health (Campbell et al., 2014) are well documented.

If markets cannot be expected to act efficiently concerning investment in early childhood development, what are the alternative policy prescriptions? Traditionally, market failure signifies a justification for government intervention in a particular sphere of economic activity. It is why large capital infrastructure projects are typically financed using taxpayer funds, why regulatory bodies exist to protect consumers against the potential consequences of free market excesses, and why such public goods as police forces, court systems, and public schools are government-financed institutions.

It should be acknowledged, however, that the breadth of this sphere of government activity is not fixed but evolves continuously over time. As government action requires either the enactment of legislation or regulatory initiatives, a ripening of political awareness remains a foundational prerequisite for these activities. Recognition of the inability of a free market to guarantee reliably a livable income for many senior citizens during a period of profound economic contraction led to the development of the Social Security Administration in the 1930s in the USA. Decades earlier, in the wake of the First World War and the Russian revolution, a similar realization that the market provided no sustainable mechanism for workers injured in the course of their jobs to receive restitution led to the enactment of the workers compensation system that we have today. More recently government programs created in the 1960s addressed acknowledged inefficiencies in the market for health insurance for elderly and poor citizens.

What each of these historical examples has in common is not that free markets suddenly failed in their ability to allocate scarce resources efficiently, but that a political realization of this inability became so irrefutable that it ultimately inspired legislation to commit the government to an activity that it had been previously unwilling to embrace. We are quite possibly at the threshold of a similar shift in thinking with respect to early childhood development. The illumination of the neurological and molecular biological mechanisms influencing the developing brain, coupled with an accumulation of persuasive empirical evidence regarding the economic benefits of investing in early child development, is shifting social perception toward an acknowledgment that the time has come to redefine public responsibility toward fostering the human capital stock of the next generation of citizens. The opportunity costs of forgoing these investments are substantial in the present and will be magnified into the future. How *politically* compelling the case has become remains the most salient question of all.

References

Aos, S., Lieb, R., Mayfield, J., Miller, M., & Pennucci, A. (2004). *Benefits and costs of prevention and early intervention programs for youth*. Olympia, WA: Washington State Institute for Public Policy.

Barnett, W. S. (1985a). Benefit-cost analysis of the perry preschool program and its policy implications. *Educational Evaluation and Policy Analysis, 7*, 333–342.

Barnett, W. S. (1985b). *The perry preschool program and its long-term effects: A benefit cost analysis*. Ypsilanti, MI: High/Scope Educational Research Foundation.

Barnett, W. S. (1993). Benefit-cost analysis of preschool education: Findings from a 25-year follow-up. *American Journal of Orthopsychiatry, 63*, 500–508.

Barnett, W. S. (2011). Effectiveness of early educational intervention. *Science, 333*, 975–978.

Barnett, W. S., & Masse, L. N. (2007). Comparative benefit-cost analysis of the Abecedarian program and its policy implications. *Economics of Education Review, 26*, 113–125.

Becker, G. S. (1975). *Human capital*. New York, NY: Columbia University Press.

Becker, G. S., & Tomes, N. (1986). Human capital and the rise and fall of families. *Journal of Labor Economics, 4*(Part 2), S1–S39.

Belfield, C. R., Nores, M., Barnett, S., & Schweinhart, L. (2006). The high/scope perry preschool program: Cost-benefit analysis using data from the age-40 follow up. *The Journal of Human Resources, 41*, 162–190.

Ben, P. Y. (1967). The production of human capital and the life cycle of earnings. *Journal of Political Economy, 75*, 352–365.

Burger, K. (2010). How does early childhood care and education affect cognitive development? An international review of the effects of early interventions for children from different social backgrounds. *Early Childhood Research Quarterly, 25*, 140–165.

Campbell, F., Conti, G., Heckman, J. J., Moon, S. H., Pinto, R., Pungello, E., & Pan, Y. (2014) Early childhood investments substantially boost adult health. *Science, 343*, 1478–1485.

Campbell, F. A., Helms, R., Sparling, J. J., & Ramey, C. T. (1998). Early childhood programs and success in school. In W. S. Barnett & S. S. Boocock (Eds.), *Early care and education for children in poverty*. New York, NY: SUNY Press.

Conti, G., & Heckman, J. J. (2012). The economics of child well-being. *Institute for the Study of Labor; IZA Discussion Paper* 6930.

Cunha, F., & Heckman, J. J. (2007). The technology of skill formation. *The American Economic Review, 97*, 31–47.

Currie, J. (2001). Early childhood education programs. *Journal of Economic Perspectives, 15*, 213–238.

Dalziel, K. M., Halliday, D., & Segal, L. (2015). Assessment of the cost-benefit literature on early childhood education for vulnerable children: what the findings mean for policy. *SAGE Open, 5*, 1–14. doi:10.1177/2158244015571637.

Davidson, R. J., & McEwen, B. S. (2012). Social influences on neuroplasticity: Stress and interventions to promote well-being. *Nature Neuroscience, 15*, 689–695.

Engle, P. L., Fernald, L. C. H., Alderman, H., Behrman, J., O'Gara, C., Yousafzai, A., et al. (2011). Strategies for reducing inequalities and improving developmental outcomes for young children in low-income and middle-income countries. *The Lancet, 378*, 1339–1353.

Gertler, P., Heckman, J. J., Pinto, R., Zanolini, A., Vermeersch, C., Walker, S., … Grantham-McGregor, S. (2013). *Labor market returns to early childhood stimulation: A 20-year follow-up to an experimental intervention in Jamaica*. NBER working paper No. 19185. Cambridge, MA: NBER.

Gold, M. R., Patrick, D. L., Torrane, G. W., Fryback, D. G., Hadorn, D. C., Kamlet, M. S, … Weinstein, M. C. (1996). Identifying and valuing outcomes. In M. R. Gold, J. E., Siegel, L. B. Russell, & M. C. Weinstein (Eds.) *Cost-effectiveness in health and medicine*. New York, NY: Oxford University Press.

Gold, M. R., Siegel, J. E., Russell, L. B., & Weinstein, M. C. (1996). *Cost-effectiveness in health and medicine*. New York, NY: Oxford University Press.

Haskins, R., & Barnett, W. S. (2010). *Investing in young children: New directions in federal preschool and early childhood policy*. New Brunswick, NJ: Rutgers University, National Institute for Early Education Research.

Heckman, J. J. (2007). The economics, technology and neuroscience of human capability formation. *PNAS, 104*, 13250–13255.

Heckman, J. J., & Masterov, D. V. (2007). The productivity argument for investing in young children. *Lecture delivered as the T.W. Schultz Award Lecture at the Allied Social Sciences Association annual meeting*. Chicago, January 5–7, 2007.

Heckman, J. J., Moon, S. H., Pinto, R., Savelyev, P. A., & Yavitz, A. (2010). The rate of return to the HighScope Perry Preschool Program. *Journal of Public Economics, 94*, 114–128.

Kilburn, M. R., & Karoly, L. A. (2008). *The economics of early childhood policy: What the dismal science has to say about investing in children*. Santa Monica, CA: The RAND Corporation.

Lee, S., Aos, S., & Miller, M. (2008). *Evidence-based programs to prevent children from entering and remaining in the child welfare system: Benefits and costs for Washington*. Olympia, WA: Washington State Institute for Public Policy.

Leibowitz, A. (1974). Home investment in children. *Journal of Political Economy, 82*, S111–S131.

Levin, H. M., & McEwan, P. J. (2001). *Cost-effectiveness analysis* (2nd ed.). Thousand Oaks, CA: Sage Publications.

Lipsey, M. W. (2003). Those confounded moderators in meta-analysis: Good, bad, and ugly. *Annals of the American Academy of Political and Social Science, 587*, 69–81.

Mankiw, N. G. (2007). *Principles of economics*. Mason, OH: Thomson Higher Education.

Marshall, A. (1997). *Principles of economics*. Amherst, NY: Prometheus Books.

Minkovitz, C. S., Hughart, N., Strobino, D., Scharfstein, D., Grason, H., Hou, W., et al. (2003). A practice-based intervention to enhance quality of care in the first three years of life: The healthy steps for young children program. *JAMA, 290*, 3081–3091.

Nores, M., Belfield, C. R., Barnett, W. S., & Schweinhart, L. (2005). Updating the economic impacts of the high/scope perry preschool program. *Educational Evaluation and Policy Analysis, 27*, 245–261.

Olds, D. L., Henderson, C. R., Tatelbaum, R., & Chamberlin, R. (1986). Improving the delivery of prenatal care and outcomes of pregnancy: A randomized trial of nurse visitation. *Pediatrics, 77*, 16–28.

Olds DL, Eckenrode J, Henderson CR Jr, Kitzman H, Powers J, Cole R, Sidora K, Morris P, Pettitt LM, Luckey D. (1997). Long-term effects of home visitation on maternal life course and child abuse and neglect. Fifteen-year follow-up of a randomized trial. *JAMA, 278*, 637–643.

Petitti, D. B. (2000). *Meta-analysis, decision analysis, and cost-effectiveness analysis: Methods for quantitative synthesis in medicine* (2nd ed.). New York, NY: Oxford University Press.

Piotrowski, C. C., Talavera, G. A., & Mayer, J. A. (2009). Healthy steps: A systematic review of a preventive practice-based model of pediatric care. *Journal of Developmental and Behavioral Pediatrics, 30*, 91–103.

Puma, M., Bell, S., Cook, R., & Heid, C. (2010). *Head start impact study final report*. Washington, DC: US Dept. HHS, Administration for Children and Families, Office of Research, Planning and Evaluation.

Reynolds, A. J. (2000). *Success in early intervention: The Chicago child-parent centers*. Lincoln, OR: University of Nebraska Press.

Reynolds, A. J., Temple, J. A., Robertson, D. L., & Mann, E. A. (2002). Age 21 cost-benefit analysis of the title I Chicago child-parent centers. *Educational Evaluation and Policy Analysis, 24*, 267–303.

Reynolds, A. J., Temple, J. A., White, B. A. B., Ou, S.-R., & Robertson, D. L. (2011). Age 26 cost-benefit analysis of the child-parent center early education program. *Child Development, 82*, 379–404.

Rolnick, A., & Grunewald, R. (2003). Early childhood development: economic development with a high public return. In Fedgazette. Retrieved from https://www.minneapolisfed.org/publications/fedgazette/early-childhood-development-economic-development-with-a-high-public-return

Schweinhart, L. J., Barnes, H. V., & Weikart, D. P. (1993). *Significant benefits: The high/scope perry preschool study through age 27*. Ypsilanti, MI: High/Scope Press.

Shonkoff, J. P., & Phillips, D. (2000). *From neurons to neighborhoods: The science of early child development*. Washington, DC: National Academy Press.

Sparling, J. J., & Lewis, I. (1979). *Learning games for the first three years: A guide to parent-child play*. New York, NY: Walker.

Sparling, J. J., & Lewis, I. (1984). *Learning games for threes and fours: A guide to adult/child play*. New York, NY: Walker.

Temple, J. A., & Reynolds, A. J. (2007). Benefits and costs of investments in preschool education: Evidence from the child-parent centers and related programs. *Economics of Education Review, 26*, 126–144.

Torrance, G. W., Siegel, J. E., & Luce, B. R. (1996). Framing and designing the cost-effectiveness analysis. In M. R. Gold, J. E. Siegel, L. B. Russell, & M. C. Weinstein (Eds.), *Cost-effectiveness in health and medicine*. New York, NY: Oxford University Press.

Yoshikawa, H. (1995). Long-term effects of early childhood programs on social outcomes and delinquency. *The Future of Children, 5*, 51–75.

Zuckerman, B., Parker, S., Kaplan-Sanoff, M., Augustyn, M., & Barth, M. C. (2004). Healthy steps: A case study of innovation in pediatric practice. *Pediatrics, 114*, 820–826.

Chapter 4
The Goodness of Fit between Evidence-Based Early Childhood Mental Health Programs and the Primary Care Setting

Dana E. Crawford and Rahil D. Briggs

Abstract With numerous evidence-based early childhood behavioral health programs, it is important to choose wisely when deciding to integrate a particular program into primary care. Most programs were designed for implementation outside of the primary care setting, and may not be a good fit, due to the unique nature of primary care (busy, episodic visits, heterogeneous populations, etc.). In this chapter, we propose five critical elements to be considered when evaluating the goodness of fit between a particular program and the primary care setting, including the evidence base, the required elements (i.e., groups, technology), educational qualifications of practitioners, the target population served, and cost. We review seven common programs, assess them according to these metrics, and present recommendations for guiding program choice.

Keywords Evidence based • Early childhood behavioral health • Primary care

In prior chapters, we have made the case for integrating early childhood behavioral health into primary care. Once the decision has been made to do so, however, a new set of questions arises, specifically about which program to consider. While there are numerous evidence-based early childhood behavioral health programs, only some have been tested within primary care. In this chapter, we make the case that, in order to determine which program is the most appropriate for a primary care setting, there needs to be a systematic manner by which programs are evaluated. We therefore present a framework for thinking precisely about this question—the "goodness of fit" between an evidence-based early childhood behavioral health program and primary care. Although some evidence-based programs have been tested in the primary care setting, others have not, and this distinction bears caution when considering adaptation. Based on our experience, we posit that there are five critical elements to examine when looking to integrate an early childhood program into primary care:

D.E. Crawford, Ph.D. (✉) • R.D. Briggs, Psy.D.
Montefiore Health System, Bronx, NY, USA
e-mail: dacrawfo@montefiore.org; rabriggs@montefiore.org

© Springer International Publishing Switzerland 2016
R.D. Briggs (ed.), *Integrated Early Childhood Behavioral Health in Primary Care*, DOI 10.1007/978-3-319-31815-8_4

1. The current evidence base for the particular program, specifically within primary care—this element may be the most important to consider, as it pertains to any evidence-based results of the particular program within primary care. We did not include individual case reports, and noted when a study was a randomized controlled trial. We report on whether there are 1–5, 6 or more, or zero reports of delivery of a certain program within primary care found in the scholarly literature.

2. Required elements: in this section, we review the required aspects of the program. For example, are groups required, which may be prohibitive to pediatric practices with limited space? Does the program have a flexible implementation strategy to accommodate the wide variability of presenting problems in primary care, or is it a "one size fits all" model? Additionally, are there any technological requirements, such as video cameras or one-way mirror? We discuss requirements in the categories of:

   (a) groups (required vs. optional),
   (b) specific population (i.e., only trauma exposed children) vs. prevention,
   (c) technology/additional equipment needed, and
   (d) prescriptive, set time frame versus flexible time frame.

3. Discipline/educational qualifications of the practitioners: we review the required training for implementing the model, both as it pertains to formal academic training and model-specific training. We note whether or not a graduate degree is required, or if undergraduate training is sufficient.

4. Cost (including initial training, ongoing consultation, training manuals and other materials, etc.): while of critical importance, this aspect proved the most difficult to reliably report. Whenever possible, we include costs based on initial and ongoing trainings, manuals, materials, and any other published cost elements (Table 4.3).

5. Target population: while some programs begin at birth, others are only evidence-based for children ages 2 and older. Such a consideration is critical when seeking to capitalize on the true preventive nature of integrated early childhood behavioral health. Additionally, some programs target parents alone (which may raise questions about childcare), whereas others are two generation in focus and include the child. We discuss whether or not programs target:

   (a) Parents only
   (b) Parents and children, beginning at infancy
   (c) Parents and children, beginning at age 2

In the following pages, we provide assessments of several early childhood programs based upon these five dimensions. At the conclusion of each, we summarize the findings with an overall evaluation of the goodness of fit between a particular program and primary care pediatrics.

We do not suggest that this is an exhaustive list of program characteristics to consider, nor do we propose that any one of these elements necessarily trumps another in importance. However, we stand by the critical need to acknowledge the unique aspects of the primary care setting when choosing a model to integrate.

Specifically, the majority of primary care practices are busy, fast moving places. An average pediatrician may see 10–15 children per afternoon, and healthcare is increasingly moving away from private, solo practitioners and toward larger group practices (Liebhaber & Grossman, 2007). Further, patients typically interact with primary care pediatrics in an episodic manner (Hagan, Shaw & Duncan, 2008), coming for well-child visits very frequently during a child's infancy, then every few months or so during toddlerhood, and annually beginning at age 3. Large pediatric practices care for a wide variety of children and families, some with significant need for intervention and others who will thrive with standard care. Thus, programs that provide for a level of flexibility, allow for the appropriate treatment of large numbers of children, and do not require daily or weekly attendance may be preferable. Cost is of course a major consideration as well, as the Triple Aim of healthcare suggests that we should strive to provide better care, improve the patient experience of care, and do it all while reducing costs (Berwick, Nolan, & Whittington, 2008).

Assessment of Programs

Method

We now turn our attention to a selection of evidence-based early childhood programs. Our selection of which programs to include was based on frequency of appearance in the literature search results, and on our own judgment regarding commonly considered programs. To attempt to ensure a national perspective on which programs are most commonly cited for inclusion in primary care, we also consulted colleagues from various regions of the country. To report on the evidence base within primary care, we conducted a literature review of the programs chosen for inclusion, with special focus on evidence-based findings within primary care pediatrics. PubMed was searched using the names of the programs and keywords: early childhood mental health, early childhood behavioral health, pediatric practice, medical home, pediatrician, and primary care. When possible, we also consulted the official website for the program. The search was conducted from March to April 2015, and again in December 2015 before the completion of the chapter in order to include up-to-date data. See Tables 4.1 and 4.2 for our findings, which will be described in more detail here. Programs are presented alphabetically.

Child–Parent Psychotherapy
childtrauma.ucsf.edu/child-parent-psychotherapy-training

Child–Parent Psychotherapy (CPP) is an intervention for families with children from birth to age 5 with behavior, attachment, and/or mental health issues due to experiencing a trauma (Child Parent Psychotherapy, 2015). The intervention aims to use the parent–/caregiver–child relationship to restore the child's sense of safety, secure attachment, and developmentally appropriate cognitive, behavioral, and social functioning (The California Evidence-Based Clearinghouse for Child Welfare, 2015a).

Evidence Specific to Implementation in Primary Care with Children 0–5: 0 Studies Found

No studies found via PubMed search

Discipline/Educational Qualifications of the Practitioners

Master's- or doctoral-level mental health provider or a supervised trainee (The California Evidence-Based Clearinghouse for Child Welfare, 2015a).

Target Population

Parents and their children, beginning at birth (The California Evidence-Based Clearinghouse for Child Welfare, 2015a).

Cost

1. Manual(s): General Training Manual = approximately $40 each
   Don't Hit My Mommy! Manual = approximately $25 each
2. Initial training: $9000–$27,000
3. Ongoing consultation: $150–$350 per hour (The California Evidence-Based Clearinghouse for Child Welfare, 2015a; National Registry of Evidence-based Programs & Practices, 2015a)

Required Elements of the Program

Groups	Specific population (S) vs. prevention (P)	Technology/additional equipment Required	Prescriptive time frame
No	S (trauma exposed)	No	Weekly sessions, for approximately 1 year

Program Evaluation Specific to Implementation In A Pediatric Primary Care Setting

There have been no studies conducted investigating CPP in a primary care setting. CPP is generally conducted weekly for approximately 1 year, which may be an inappropriately lengthy treatment approach in a primary care setting. Furthermore, CPP is designed to treat children exposed to trauma, which excludes the majority of children seen within a primary care setting.

Circle of Security Parenting (COS-P) www.circleofsecurity.net

The COS program is a visually based approach (i.e., one that uses visual aids such as videos, magnets, handouts, and photographs) to parent training aimed at increasing caregivers' awareness of children's needs. With increased awareness, caregivers become more mindful and less reactive, respond more effectively to children's needs, and reduce problematic attachment patterns that may have been passed down through generations. The program is based in attachment theory and is used in a variety of settings such as group, family therapy, individual therapy, and home visitation. Regardless of the format, the consistent themes are teaching basics of attachment theory, improving parent skills through increasing parent sensitivity and responsiveness to children's needs, reflective dialogue, and exploring defensive mechanisms with parents. The COS Program offers six types of training. The three types of training most relevant to the primary care setting are the Introductory Training, Parenting Training, and Intensive Training. At the time of this review, the Introductory Training was not available. The Parenting Training is a 4-day seminar and DVD parent education program offering the core components of the COS protocol. The Intensive Training offers tools for competency in evaluation and treatment planning for the COS protocol. The following is a review of the Parent Training and DVD program and the Intensive Training (Circle of Security, 2015).

Evidence Findings Specific to Implementation In Primary Care with Children 0–5: 0 Studies Found

No studies found

Discipline/Educational Qualifications of the Practitioners Delivering the Program

Supervisors: Graduate degree, license required, and must have completed the basic 10-day intensive training and received at least 1 year of supervision from one of the Circle of Security originators (The California Evidence-Based Clearinghouse for Child Welfare 2015b).

Practitioners: Undergraduate degree *and* in the field of providing parent education.

Target Population

Parents and their children, beginning at birth (The California Evidence-Based Clearinghouse for Child Welfare 2015b).

Cost

1. Manual(s): approximately $40
2. Initial training: $1000 (Parent Training & DVD)/$2600 (Intensive Training), plus required $200 certification fee
3. Ongoing consultation: The availability of/cost of consultation was not listed on the website, therefore is unknown (Circle of Security, 2015)

Required Elements of the Program

Groups?	Specific population (S) vs. prevention (P)	Technology/additional equipment Required	Prescriptive time frame
Optional	P	Yes (device to play DVD)	8- or 20-week courses of treatment

Program Evaluation Specific to Implementation in a Pediatric Primary Care Setting

There have been no studies conducted investigating Circle of Security in a primary care setting. The majority of the evidence-based reports have used a group-based approach, which may present challenges in the primary care setting. Additionally, although the COS literature indicates that the initial assessment of the parent–child dyad results in an individualized plan for the dyad, the intervention is still a prescriptive 90 min, 8- or 20-week course focused on the content of the DVD. Depending on the dyad, a 90 min, 8- or 20-week course may or may not be necessary, and this may be an area of weakness for a primary care setting with a heterogeneous patient population.

Healthy Steps
www.healthysteps.org

Healthy Steps is an initiative targeted at promoting the cognitive, physical, and emotional development of children between birth to 3 years within a pediatric or family medicine setting. The Healthy Steps Specialist (HSS) serves as the primary child development resource for families and works collaboratively with pediatric practitioners. The HSS provides enhanced well-child care (conducting well-child office appointments jointly or sequentially with the pediatric practitioner), a child development telephone information line, home visits, informational materials, child development screening and family health checkups, parent groups, and links to community resources. The intensity of services is customized to the family (Healthy Steps, 2015).

Evidence Findings Specific to Implementation in Primary Care with Children 0–5: 6+

There are numerous studies (>20) pointing to the efficacy of Healthy Steps, a program that was designed exclusively for delivery within the primary care setting. Space limitations prohibit us from reviewing all of the published studies here. The original Healthy Steps evaluation was a randomized controlled trial and found positive outcomes related to the quality of early childhood healthcare and parenting practices (Minkovitz et al., 2003). Related to the quality of care, findings revealed that, for example, families received ≥4 Healthy Steps-related services or discussed >6 anticipatory guidance topics, families were satisfied with care provided, children received timely well-child visits and vaccinations, and families remained at the practice for ≥20 months. Parenting outcomes included response to child misbehavior (e.g., reduced use of severe discipline) and practices to promote child development and safety (e.g., mothers at risk for depression discussed their sadness with someone at the practice).

Other studies have generally agreed with these findings, and have also focused on child outcomes, including increased likelihood of secure attachments, reduced incidence of behavior problems (Caughy, Huang, Miller & Genevro, 2004), and improved social emotional development (Briggs et al., 2014). Procedural outcomes have also been shown, related to, for example, increased incidence of breastfeeding and reading to children in Healthy Steps families (Johnston, Huebner, Tyll, Barlow & Thompson, 2004).

Finally, a systematic review of Healthy Steps was conducted by Piotrowski et al. (Piotrowski, Talavera, & Mayer, 2009) and results indicated that the Healthy Steps program has been rigorously evaluated and shown to be effective in preventing negative child and parent outcomes and enhancing positive outcomes.

Discipline/Educational Qualifications of the Practitioners Delivering the Program

Undergraduate with significant experience or graduate degree in relevant field (Healthy Steps, 2015).

Target Population

Parents and children, beginning at birth (some programs offer enrollment prenatally) (Healthy Steps, 2015).

Cost

1. Manual(s): "Getting Started Package": $100
2. Initial training: $12,000–$18,000
3. Ongoing consultation: included
4. Average cost per family per year is approximately $412.95/family (Healthy Steps, 2015)

Required Elements of the Program

Groups?	Specific population (S) vs. prevention (P)	Technology/additional equipment Required	Prescriptive time frame
Optional	P	No	Flexible

Program Evaluation Specific to Implementation in a Pediatric Primary Care Setting

Healthy Steps (HS) was designed specifically to address, in a prospective/preemptive manner, the behavioral and developmental support needs of families bringing their young children to pediatric care settings. The Healthy Steps program has been rigorously evaluated and shown to be effective in preventing negative child and parent outcomes and enhancing positive outcomes. Research has indicated that families who participate in HS are more satisfied with care, more likely to receive needed anticipatory guidance, have increased odds of remaining at the original practice, have reduced odds of using severe discipline, increased odds of often/almost always negotiating with their child, greater odds of reporting a clinical or borderline concern regarding their child's behavior, and greater odds of engaging in developmentally appropriate parenting. The Healthy Steps program provides clear benefit through early screening, family-centered care, and evidence-based anticipatory guidance in primary care settings. As it was specifically designed for integration into primary care, no specific limitations emerge. As a note, the authors are members of a healthcare system that employs Healthy Steps.

Incredible Years
www.incredibleyears.com

The Incredible Years (IY) Series is a comprehensive group-based program for parents, teachers, and children aimed at preventing, reducing, and treating behavioral, social, and emotional problems for children ages birth to 12 years. The parent programs target key developmental stages: IY Baby Program (0–12 months), IY Toddler Basic Program (1–3 years), IY Preschool Basic (3–6 years), IY School Age Basic (6–12 years), and Advanced Parenting Program (4–12 years) (focuses on parent interpersonal problems such as depression and anger management). Additionally, there are four adjunct parent programs: Well-Baby Prevention Program, Attentive Parenting Prevention Program, Autism Spectrum and Language Delays Program, and the School Readiness Program. There are two child programs using the Dinosaur School Social Emotional Skills and Problem Solving Curriculum: Small Group Dinosaur Child Treatment Program (ages 4–8 years) and Classroom Dinosaur Prevention Program (ages 3–8 years). Finally, there are two teacher programs: Teacher Classroom Management Program for teachers of children ages 3–8 years, and Incredible Beginnings Program, for teachers and child care providers of children ages 1–5 years (The Incredible Years® Parent, Teacher and Child Programs Fact Sheet, www.incredibleyears.com). The program is based on video modeling, observational and experiential learning, rehearsal and practice, individual goal setting, self-management, self-reflection, and cognitive self-control (The Incredible Years, 2015).

Evidence Findings Specific to Implementation in Primary Care with Children 0–5: 1–5 Studies

The PubMed literature search revealed four studies reporting on the implementation of Incredible Years in pediatric primary care, and they tend to show improvements in parenting practices and child behavior (McMenamy, Sheldrick, & Perrin, 2011; Perrin, Sheldrick, McMenamy, Henson, & Carter, 2014; Reedtz, Handegard, &

Morch, 2011). One study failed to find effect unless dosage was considered, and reported that at least seven to nine sessions of Incredible Years were necessary to show positive outcomes in child behavior (Lavigne et al., 2008).

Discipline/Educational Qualifications of the Practitioners Delivering the Program

Treatment Model At least 1 group leader must be Master's level or higher in a relevant field
Prevention Model Bachelor level with developmental training (The Incredible Years, 2015).

Target Population

Parents, children, and teachers beginning at birth (The Incredible Years, 2015).

Cost

1. Manual: General Manual specific to selected series = $20–40 each (required)

   The Incredible Years: A Troubleshooting Guide (recommended) = $20
   Program materials = $1150–$1895 (depending on series selected)
   Training Handouts = $20 each (required)

2. Initial Training: $400–$500 per participant per day, plus travel to training site or onsite training for $1650–$2000 per day (3+ days required), plus $450 certification fee

3. Ongoing consultation: 2 h/month at $150/h (optional) (National Registry of Evidence-based Programs and Practices, 2015b)

Required Elements of the Program

Groups?	Specific population (S) vs. prevention (P)	Technology/additional equipment Required	Prescriptive time frame
Yes	Treatment model = S (children with behavioral problems)	DVD, books, handouts	Weekly, 2-h sessions, for 14–22 weeks per cohort
	Prevention model = P		

Program Evaluation Specific to Implementation in a Pediatric Primary Care Setting

Incredible Years provides group-based comprehensive services for parents, teachers, and children aimed at preventing, reducing, and treating behavioral, social, and emotional problems for children ages 2–12 years. Findings have shown improvements in parenting practices and child behavior. However, the structure of the program requires groups, and it may be challenging to implement a 14-week group, conducted by two providers, in a primary care setting. Finally, the Incredible Years program does not provide individualized services based on patient needs, which may be an area of weakness for a primary care setting.

Parent–Child Interaction Therapy
www.pcit.org

Parent–Child Interaction Therapy (PCIT) is a treatment program for young children with behavioral problems that place emphasis on improving the quality of the parent–child relationship and changing parent–child interaction patterns. PCIT was developed for children ages 2–7 years with externalizing behavior disorders. In PCIT, parents are taught specific skills to establish or strengthen a nurturing and secure relationship with their child while encouraging prosocial behavior and discouraging negative behavior. Ideally, during coaching sessions, the therapist observes the interaction from behind a one-way mirror and provides guidance to the parent through a "bug-in-the-ear" hearing device. PCIT is generally administered in 15 weekly, 1-h sessions in an outpatient clinic by a licensed mental health professional with experience working with children and families (National Registry of Evidence-based Programs and Practices 2015c).

Evidence Findings Specific to Implementation in Primary Care with Children 0–5: 1 Study

We found one study to report on the implementation of PCIT within primary care. Berkovits et al. (2010) compared two abbreviated versions of PCIT within primary care for preschool-aged children in pediatric primary care with subclinical behavior problems. Children either received a 4-session group preventive intervention called Primary Care PCIT (PC-PCIT); or (b) written materials describing basic steps of PCIT and guidelines for practice, called PCIT Anticipatory Guidance (PCIT-AG). Although both groups showed decreased child behavior problems and ineffective parenting techniques, there was no difference between the two versions. Decreases in child problem behaviors and ineffective parenting strategies and increases in parental feelings of control were not significantly different between versions at post-intervention or 6-month follow-up.

Discipline/Educational Qualifications of the Practitioners Delivering the Program

Master's degree with license or a psychology doctoral student who has completed the third year of training and is conducting clinical work under the supervision of a licensed mental health provider (Parent-Child Interaction Therapy, 2015).

Target Population

Parents and children, beginning at child age 2, child with disruptive behaviors (Parent Child Interaction Therapy, 2015).

Cost

1. Manual: Included in training costs
2. Initial training $4000 per person, plus $200 certification fee
3. Ongoing consultation: $1000 per year, per trainee (University of Colorado Boulder Institute of Behavioral Science, 2015a)

Required Elements of the Program

Groups?	Specific population (S) vs. prevention (P)	Technology/additional equipment Required	Prescriptive time frame
Optional	S—children with behavioral problems	One-way mirror, observation room, or bug in the ear technology	Weekly, 1-h sessions, for 15 weeks

Program Evaluation Specific to Implementation in a Pediatric Primary Care Setting

PCIT has extensive research demonstrating its effectiveness in mental health clinics; however, there has been only one published study examining its effectiveness in the primary care setting, and this protocol did not use the (required) one-way mirror. The study specifically examined the effectiveness of six groups, with 2–4 mother–child dyads per group, which met for 4 weekly 1½ h sessions. All of the children in this study had only mild behavioral issues. Conducting a group for 1½ h per week in a primary care setting may not be feasible, depending on space limitations. The program age range is also a limitation, as it is not evidence based for children under age 2.

Triple P Parenting
www.triplep.net/glo-en/home

The Triple P—Positive Parenting System is a five-level prevention and treatment program for behavioral and emotional problems in children and adolescents, based on social learning, cognitive behavioral, and developmental theories. Triple P aims to teach parents the skills they need to be competent in effectively managing family issues, aims for children to develop emotional self-regulation, and for parents to be effective problem-solvers. Practitioners use seminars, parent skills-training sessions, and individual consultations to guide parents, with the aim of preventing dysfunctional parenting and child maltreatment. Services are tailored to the severity of the family's dysfunction and/or the child's behavioral problems and range from one to ten or more sessions. Sessions are conducted in a variety of settings (e.g., healthcare, preschools, elementary schools, mental health, social services).

The five levels of intervention represent stepped up care with increasing intensity. Each of the five levels is defined by the intensity of intervention, choice of delivery method, and severity of behavioral symptoms. Within the five levels, primary care focused interventions occur at levels 2 and 3. In level 2, Brief Primary Care Triple P services are offered, and are usually of a one-time nature, brief, and targeting a specific issue. Level 3 includes Primary Care Triple P services, which are approximately four brief face to face or telephone interventions, appropriate for mild and specific behavioral concerns (Triple P Parenting, 2015).

Triple P Parenting Evidence Findings Specific to Implementation In Primary Care with Children 0–5: 6+

The PubMed search revealed seven reports on integrating Triple P into primary care, and the results are inconsistent. Turner and Sanders (2006) investigated a brief (three to four sessions) Triple P program, delivered in primary care, and found lower levels of targeted child behavior problems, dysfunctional parenting, and reduced parental anxiety and stress in comparison to wait-listed parents at post-assessment. Boyle et al. (2010) reported lower levels of child disruptive behavior, maintained over time, and higher parental self-efficacy reports. However, there was no statistically significant effect on observed parenting practices. While McConnell et al. (2012) reported that parents who participated in Triple P Primary Care endorsed higher levels of satisfaction regarding their role, no significant difference was found (when comparing to care as usual) related to parenting stress, positive interaction, family functioning, or child problem behaviors. Finally, Schappin et al. (2014) found no impact of Primary Care Triple P on parenting skills for parents of NICU graduates, and Spijkers et al. (2013) reported a lack of significant findings when assessing the impact of Primary Care Triple P for parents of children with mild behavioral problems.

Two studies have examined the implementation process of Primary Care Triple P. In their examination of factors affecting the implementation of Primary Care Triple P, Turner et al. (2011) found lack of compatibility at the program and workplace level (e.g., lack of clients, program not appropriate for clients, limitations of normal work hours, lack of supervision) and difficulty of implementation (e.g., difficulties with time management, engaging clients, setting goals) were barriers to implementation. On the other hand, they found that flexibility (e.g., ability to tailor to individual needs) and training/preparation factors (e.g., knowledge and skills in behavioral family interventions and behavior change) supported implementation. McCormick et al. (2014) reported that pediatric residents trained in Primary Care Triple P improved their parenting consultation skills, and parents visiting these residents increased their positive disciplinary strategies compared to parents visiting control residents. There were no differences found for child behavior or parenting sense of confidence.

Discipline/Educational Qualifications of the Practitioners Delivering the Program

Triple P Trainers master's degree or higher required
Triple P Providers paraprofessionals or undergraduate (Triple P Parenting, 2015).

Target Population

Parents of children beginning at birth, children not included (Triple P Parenting, 2015).

Cost

1. Manual: Included in training costs
2. Initial Training: Primary Care Triple P = $23,555
3. Ongoing Consultation: Included in training costs (University of Colorado Boulder Institute of Behavioral Science, 2015b)

Required Elements of the Program

Groups?	Specific population (S) vs. prevention (P)	Technology/additional equipment Required	Prescriptive time frame
Optional	S—Primary care models are focused on parents with concerns regarding child development/behavior	Yes (device to play DVD)	Approximately four individual consultations of between 15 and 30 min

Program Evaluation Specific to Implementation in a Pediatric Primary Care Setting

The diversity of intervention formats (e.g., seminars, parent skills-training sessions, and individual consultations), the flexibility to adapt interventions to the severity of the family's level of needs, and the evidence-based age range extending down to birth are three of the greatest strengths of the Triple P—Positive Parenting System for integration into primary care. Furthermore, the Triple P extension program, Primary Care Triple P, has been specifically designed for implementation in primary care settings. However, it should be noted that Primary Care Triple P is designed to be implemented by primary care practitioners (nursing, allied health, education, and medical). Additionally, although specifically designed for the primary care setting, the literature suggests some barriers to implementation.

Video Interaction Project
www.childrenofbellevue.org/video-interaction-project

Video Interaction Project (VIP) is a relationship-based intervention that coincides with pediatric well visits from birth to 5 years of age. The interactions between mother–child dyads are recorded, with the goal of reinforcing interactional strengths. More specifically, the interventionist makes video recordings of parents and their child playing and then uses the videos, via shared review, to increase the parents' understanding of their interactions and identify ways to improve. Toys and books that have been specifically selected to promote parent–child engagement and child development are given to parents to take home (Video Interaction Project, 2015).

Evidence Findings Specific to Implementation in Primary Care with Children 0–5: 1–5 Studies

Like Healthy Steps, VIP was designed exclusively for inclusion into primary care visits. However, it has not yet been expanded beyond the original team, and all results come from the founder of the program and his colleagues. Mendelsohn et al. (2005) originally reported on their randomized controlled trial to assess the impact of (VIP) on cognitive and language development at age 21 months. Results differed depending on the level of maternal education; VIP was found to have a moderate impact on children whose mothers had between seventh and 11th grade education (approximately 0.75 SD for cognitive development, 0.5 SD for expressive language), but little impact on children whose mothers had sixth grade or lower education. In 2007, they followed up with a report of the children at 33 months and found improved parenting practices and lower levels of parenting stress. At 33 months, VIP children were more likely to have normal cognitive development and less likely to have developmental delays, compared to controls. The team has also compared VIP to a second intervention called Building Blocks [BB], which provided written materials to parents. In this evaluation (2011), the VIP group and the BB group showed similar results.

Discipline/Educational Qualifications of the Practitioners Delivering the Program

No specific qualifications are listed (Video Interaction Project, 2015).

Target Population

Parents and children, beginning at birth (Video Interaction Project, 2015).

Cost (Training, Materials, Supervision Costs, Any Data Re: Cost Per Child Served)

The price of the VIP program could not be obtained (Video Interaction Project, 2015).

Required Elements of the Program

Groups?	Specific population (S) vs. prevention (P)	Technology/additional equipment Required	Prescriptive time frame
Not required	P	Video recording and playback technology; toy or book given out each visit; video tape given out each visit	Flexible

Program Evaluation Specific to Implementation in a Pediatric Primary Care Setting

VIP uses video recordings to increase parents understanding of their parent–child interactions and identify ways to improve these interactions. VIP coincides with pediatric well visits and is designed for delivery within the primary care setting.

Evidence (at this point only published by the originators of the program) suggests that VIP is associated with lower levels of parenting stress and improved developmental outcomes for children. However, the program may present significant limitations for parents that are against being video recorded (e.g., undocumented parents, religious reasons, discomfort), and for practices who don't wish to incur the burden and expense of maintaining the necessary video equipment. Additional costs include toys and books for parents to take home. Finally, the program is relatively new and has not yet outlined an approach to dissemination and replication.

Conclusion

The process of determining the best evidence-based program to implement in any setting can be challenging. Obtaining information on the effectiveness of evidence-based programs to be implemented in primary care settings has been a difficult task due to underdeveloped websites, lack of concrete details about specific aspects of the program, and limited research. After conducting a thorough review, Healthy Steps emerges as the most well-studied program that attends to the unique needs of the primary care setting, as it was developed with the primary care setting in mind. Triple P Parenting's Primary Care program also shows promise, with diversity of intervention formats and flexible intervention options. However, it is notable that the research indicates that there are compatibility and implementation barriers (e.g., difficulties with time management, engaging clients, setting goals) with the Primary Care program. Although VIP was also designed for the primary care setting, it has not been replicated beyond the original team, and thus shows less evidence, has no information re: cost and training, etc. The other programs reviewed in this chapter, while certainly of excellent caliber when offered in the manner they were designed, may offer primary care modifications and yet would likely present barriers in primary care settings. For instance, some programs require groups, video recording, numerous providers, numerous sessions, or lack a clear implementation structure. All of these factors would be noteworthy in the fast paced primary care setting. Additionally, many programs fail to demonstrate evidence-based findings for children under age 2. As discussed elsewhere in this volume, it is critical to intervene with children as early as possible, and a good fit for primary care early childhood programming should start at birth. We hope that our efforts in this chapter will help to guide thoughtful implementation of primary care early childhood behavioral health programs (Table 4.3).

Table 4.1 Summary chart of all programs

Intervention	Target population (2-gen = parent/ child)	Groups required?	Specific population (S) vs. prevention (P)	Technology or additional equipment required	Prescriptive time frame	Master's degree required?	# Studies re: primary care (0, 1–5, 6+)
Child–Parent Psychotherapy	Starts at birth, 2-gen	No	S (trauma exposed)	No	Weekly sessions, for approximately 1 year	Yes, or under supervision	0
Circle of Security	Starts at birth, 2-gen	Optional	P	Yes (device to play DVD)	8- or 20-week courses	Yes, for supervisors; No, for practitioners	0
Healthy Steps	Starts at birth or prenatally, 2-gen	Optional	P	No	No	No	6+
Incredible Years	Starts at birth, 2-gen	Yes	P and S (behavior problems)	Yes (device to play DVD)	14–22 weekly sessions	Yes, for intervention; No, for prevention	1–5
Parent–Child Interaction Therapy (PCIT)	Starts at age 2, 2-gen	Optional	S (behavior problems)	Yes (One-way mirror, observation room, or bug in the ear technology)	15 weeks	Yes, or under supervision	1–5
Triple P Parenting— Primary Care	Starts at birth, parents only	Optional	S (parents with concerns re: child dev/ behavior)	Yes (device to play DVD)	Approximately four brief individual consultations	Yes, for trainers; No for providers	6+
Video Interaction Project (VIP)	Starts at birth, 2-gen	No	P	Yes (Video recording/ playback technology; toy or book given each visit; video tape given each visit)	No	Unknown	1–5

Table 4.2 Evidence-based early childhood programs and primary care

Program name	Evidence-based findings	Evidence in primary care with children 0–5 years	Discipline/educational qualifications of the practitioners	Target population	Cost (training, materials, supervision costs, any data re: cost per child served)	Required elements of the program
Child–Parent Psychotherapy (CPP)	Toth, Maughan, Manly, Spagnola, and Cicchetti (2002) A comparison study of the preschooler–parent psychotherapy (PPP), psychoeducational home visitation (PHV) vs. community standard (CS) revealed that PPP maltreated preschoolers had more declines in maladaptive maternal representations, decreases in negative self-representations, and more positive mother–child relationship expectations over time than PHV or CS Lieberman, Ippen, and Van Horn (2006) Random assignment comparison study of CPP vs. case management plus community referral indicated decreased behavioral problems and maternal distress; however, there were no significant changes in maternal symptoms Toth, Rogosch, Manly, and Cicchetti (2006) Attachment changed from insecure to secure significantly more (54.3 %) in toddlers of depressed mothers who received Toddler-PP than in toddlers of depressed mothers who received other mental health treatment (7.4 %)	No studies found	Master's- or doctoral-level mental health provider or a supervised trainee	Birth through age 5 who have experienced at least one traumatic event and as a result, are experiencing behavior, attachment, and/or mental health problems	1. Manual(s): General Training Manual =approximately $40 each Don't Hit My Mommy! Manual = approximately $25 each 2. Initial training: $9000–$27,000 3. Ongoing consultation: $150–$350 per hour (The California Evidence-Based Clearinghouse for Child Welfare 2015a; National Registry of Evidence-based Programs & Practices, 2015a)	Focus on the parent–child relationship Focus on safety Affect regulation Reciprocity in relationships Focus on the traumatic event Continuity of daily living Reflective supervision

Program name	Evidence-based findings	Evidence in primary care with children 0–5 years	Discipline/educational qualifications of the practitioners	Target population	Cost (training, materials, supervision costs, any data re: cost per child served)	Required elements of the program
	Dowell and Ogles (2010) Comparison meta-analytic review of individual child treatment vs. parent–child/family therapy treatment groups indicated treatments that involve parents/family are moderately more effective					
Circle Of Security (COS)	Hoffman, et al. (2006) In a pre-post study of 65 toddler/preschooler–caregiver dyads insecure attachments decreased from 80 % to 46%. In particular, disorganized attachment classifications decreased from 60 % to 25 % Cassidy et al. (2011) COS—Home Visiting Intervention significantly reduced the risk of insecure attachment in irritable newborns and their economically stressed mothers	No studies found	Undergraduate degree and in the field of providing parent education. Supervisors are licensed mental health providers who have completed the basic 10-day intensive training, and received at least one year of supervision from one of the Circle of Security originators (www.circleofsecurity.org)	For parents or caregivers of children ages 0–5 years	1. Manual(s): approximately $40 2. Initial training: $1000 (Parent Training & DVD) or $2600 (Intensive Training), plus required $200 certification fee 3. Ongoing consultation: The availability of/cost of consultation was not listed on the website, therefore is unknown (Circle of Security, 2015)	There is a sequence of five overarching therapeutic goals used for all parents: 1. Create a holding environment 2. Teach attachment theory in a user-friendly manner 3. Help parents develop observation skills 4. Engage in reflective dialogue between therapist and parent (central dynamic for change) 5. Support parents' empathic shift from defensive process to empathy for their children

(continued)

Table 4.2 (continued)

Program name	Evidence-based findings	Evidence in primary care with children 0–5 years	Discipline/educational qualifications of the practitioners	Target population	Cost (training, materials, supervision costs, any data re: cost per child served)	Required elements of the program
Healthy Steps	HS is a primary care based intervention; therefore, the research conducted on its effectiveness has been in a primary care setting (see next column)	Johnston et al. (2004) In a concurrent comparison study of 5 primary care clinics, the HS intervention was associated with timely well-child care, immunization rates, breastfeeding, television viewing, injury prevention, and discipline strategies. Additionally, prenatal HS was associated with larger expressive vocabularies at age 24 months Minkovitz et al. (2007) At 5.5 years evaluation HS families were more satisfied with care, more likely to receive needed anticipatory guidance, more likely to obtain treatment from original pediatric practice, less likely to use severe discipline, more likely to negotiating with the child, and had greater odds of reporting a clinical or borderline concern regarding their child's behavior Piotrowski et al. (2009) Systematic evaluation of rigorous HS studies indicated HS is effective in preventing negative child and parent outcomes and enhancing positive outcomes and provides clear cost benefits	Undergraduate with significant experience, or graduate	Parents and their children from birth to age 3	1. Manual(s): "Getting Started Package": $100 2. Initial training: $12,000–$18,000 3. Ongoing consultation: included 4. Average cost per family per year is approximately $412.95/family. (Healthy Steps, 2015)	Source: www. healthysteps.org Offer at a minimum these Healthy Steps components: home visits, child development checkups (including formal developmental screen), child development telephone information line, and Healthy Steps parent information materials

Program name	Evidence-based findings	Evidence in primary care with children 0–5 years	Discipline/educational qualifications of the practitioners	Target population	Cost (training, materials, supervision costs; any data re: cost per child served)	Required elements of the program
		Briggs et al. (2014) We describe a Healthy Steps (HS) program and the moderating effect of this program on the relationship between reported caregiver childhood trauma and child social–emotional development. In a quasi-experimental, longitudinal design, we determined the relationship between maternal report of childhood trauma and child social–emotional development on the Ages and Stages Questionnaires: Social–Emotional (ASQ:SE) at 36 months, adjusting for covariates, and tested for a moderating effect of participation in HS on this relationship. One hundred twenty-four children were assessed at 36 months. Children of mothers with childhood trauma had higher (worse) ASQ:SE mean scores than children of mothers without childhood trauma (75.9 vs. 35.9; $p < .0001$). Differences in adjusted mean ASQ:SE scores between children of mothers with and without childhood trauma were more apparent in the comparison group (90.4 vs. 28.3) than in HS (44.5 vs. 28.2; $p < .001$). Caregiver experiences of childhood trauma are related to deficits in social–emotional development in their 3-year-old children. HS, with a focus on caregiver trauma and child social–emotional development, may serve as a moderator of this association				

(continued)

Table 4.2 (continued)

Program name	Evidence-based findings	Evidence in primary care with children 0–5 years	Discipline/educational qualifications of the practitioners	Target population	Cost (training, materials, supervision costs, any data re: cost per child served)	Required elements of the program
Incredible Years (IY)	Webster-Stratton, Reid, and Beauchaine (2011) Comparison of Incredible Years intervention or the wait-list control group indicated children's externalizing, hyperactivity, inattentive and oppositional behaviors decreased and emotion regulation, social competence, emotional vocabulary, and problem-solving abilities increased. Observations revealed mothers increased praise and coaching, decreased critical statements, and children's total deviant behaviors decreased	Lavigne et al. (2008) Comparison of 12-session IY program led by primary care nurses vs. clinical psychologists vs. providing parents with only the companion book to the treatment program IY revealed improvement across posttreatment and 12-month follow-up for all groups, but no overall treatment group effects McMenamy et al. (2011) IY was delivered in 10-week group parenting programs, delivered in two primary care sites. Mothers reported improvements in their parenting skills, and in the behavioral problems of their children Reedtz et al. (2011) In a randomized controlled trial (RCT) in a primary care setting of IY parents had reductions in harsh parenting, increased positive parenting, and increased sense of competence Perrin et al. (2014) Comparison of parents from 11 pediatric practices participating in 10-week IY group vs. to a waiting list (WL) indicated decrease in parent self-reports of negative parenting behaviors and child disruptive behaviors. No differences were noted for the WL group	Treatment Model: At least 1 group leader must be Master's level or higher; however, it is recommended both leaders are Master's level or higher Prevention Model: Bachelor level with developmental training	Parents and children, beginning at birth	1. Manual: General Manual specific to selected series = $20–40 each (required) The Incredible Years: A Troubleshooting Guide (recommended) = $20 Program materials = $1150–$1895 (depending on series selected) Training Handouts = $20 each (required) 2. Initial Training: $400–$500 per participant per day, plus travel to training site or onsite training for $1650–$2000 per day (3+ days required), plus $450 certification fee 3. Ongoing consultation: 2 h/month at $150/h (optional) (National Registry of Evidence-based Programs and Practices 2015b)	Each of the types of programs consists of videotapes, comprehensive facilitator manuals, books, take-home assignments, and handouts. It is recommended that all group participants (parents, teachers, children) have their own individual books and that facilitators have their own manuals. Each group should have two group leaders

Program name	Evidence-based findings	Evidence in primary care with children 0–5 years	Discipline/educational qualifications of the practitioners	Target population	Cost (training, materials, supervision costs, any data re: cost per child served)	Required elements of the program
Parent–Child Interaction Therapy (PCIT)	Schuhmann, Foote, Eyberg, Boggs, and Algina (1998) Comparison of PCIT vs. wait-list control indicated parents in the PCIT group reported increased child compliance with parental commands, decreased parenting stress, and increased internal locus of control. Wait-list control group remained unchanged Chaffin et al. (2004) Participants were assigned to a PCIT group, a PCIT plus individualized enhanced services (EPCIT) group, or a standardized community-based parenting group. The PCIT group and the EPCIT group revealed decreases in negative parental behaviors. There was no change in the community-based parenting group Nixon (2001) A comparison of standard PCIT, abbreviated PCIT, and wait-list control (WL) indicated decrease in parent-reported externalizing behavior and parental stress and improved discipline practices in both PCIT groups compared with the WL group. Immediately after the intervention, standard PCIT suggested a superior effect, however at 6-month follow-up, both PCIT were comparable	Berkovits, O'Brien, Carter, and Eyberg (2010) Comparison of group PCIT vs. written materials revealed decreases in child problem behaviors and ineffective parenting strategies, and increases in parental feelings of control, across both versions of PCIT	Master's degree with license or a psychology doctoral student who has completed the third year of training and is conducting clinical work under the supervision of a licensed mental health provider	Parents and children, beginning at child age 2	1. Manual: Included in training costs 2. Initial training $4000 per person, plus $200 certification fee 3. Ongoing consultation: $1000 per year, per trainee (University of Colorado Boulder Institute of Behavioral Science, 2015a)	Use of standardized assessment instruments to guide treatment (e.g., Eyberg Child Behavior Inventory, Dyadic Parent–child Interaction Coding System-III) Inclusion of both the Child Directed Interaction and Parent Directed Interaction phases of treatment Coaching of parents in live interactions with their children for the majority of non-didactic sessions Coding of parent–child interactions almost every coaching session Assignment of homework between sessions

(continued)

Table 4.2 (continued)

Program name	Evidence-based findings	Evidence in primary care with children 0–5 years	Discipline/educational qualifications of the practitioners	Target population	Cost (training, materials, supervision costs, any data re: cost per child served)	Required elements of the program
	Boggs et al. (2005) A longitudinal comparison of 23 completers and 23 study dropouts completers of PCIT treatment indicated consistently better long-term outcomes for those who completed treatment than for study dropouts					
The Triple P—Positive Parenting Program	Markie-Dadds and Sanders (2006) Comparison of Self-directed Triple P group (SD) vs. wait-list group (WL). At 6-month follow-up, mothers in the SD group reported significantly less child behavior problems, less use of dysfunctional discipline strategies, and greater parenting competence than mothers in the WL group. There was no significant difference in either group on measures of parental adjustment Morawska and Sanders (2006) Comparison of self-administered alone or self-administered plus brief therapist telephone assistance indicated that families who received minimal therapist assistance made more clinically significant gains compared with families who completed the program with no therapist assistance	Turner and Sanders (2006) A comparison of brief 3- to 4-session Primary Care Triple P (PCTP) with preschool-aged children in a primary care setting vs. a wait-list control condition. Parents who received PCTP reported significantly lower levels of targeted child behavior problems, dysfunctional parenting, and reduced parental anxiety and stress at post-assessment and 6-month follow-up Boyle et al. (2010) Primary Care Triple P was delivered to 9 families with a total of 10 children aged between 3 and 7 years. Post-intervention observations of parent–child interaction in the home revealed lower levels of child disruptive behavior, and these observations were corroborated by parental report McConnell, Breitkreuz, and Savage (2012) In a comparison of levels 2 and 3 of Triple P system (designed for primary care settings) vs. service-as-usual, there was no significant difference found between Triple P and service-as-usual groups on any secondary outcome measures including parenting stress, positive interaction, family functioning and child problem behaviors	Triple P Trainers are masters- or doctorate-level professionals Triple P Providers are paraprofessionals or undergraduates who are actively involved in "hands-on" roles working with parents, children, and teens (e.g., home health visitors, promoters, and parent partners). It is expected that these particular practitioners have developed some knowledge of child/adolescent development and/or have experience working with families and also have access to adequate clinical supervision and support on a regular basis	Triple P is delivered to parents of children, beginning at birth	1. Manual: Included in training costs 2. Initial Training: Primary Care Triple P=$23,555 3. Ongoing Consultation: Included in training costs (University of Colorado Boulder Institute of Behavioral Science, 2015b)	The 5 core principles of positive parenting that are integrated throughout the multi-level Triple P system to promote social competence and emotion self-regulation in children are: (1) ensuring a safe, engaging environment, (2) promoting a positive learning environment, (3) using assertive discipline, (4) maintaining reasonable expectations, and (5) taking care of oneself as a parent

Program name	Evidence-based findings	Evidence in primary care with children 0–5 years	Discipline/educational qualifications of the practitioners	Target population	Cost (training, materials, supervision costs, any data re: cost per child served)	Required elements of the program
	Sanders, Kirby, Tellegen, and Day (2014) A systematic and meta-analysis of 101 studies over a 33-year period with 16,099 families. Short-term and long-term effects of Triple P include children's social, emotional, and behavioral outcomes; parenting practices; parenting satisfaction and efficacy; parental adjustment; parental relationship; child observational data; and parent observational data. Positive results were found on each level of the Triple P system in promoting child, parent, and family well-being	Spijkers, Jansen, and Reijneveld (2013) In a comparison of Primary Care Triple P (PCTP) program compared with care as usual (UC) for parents of children with mild psychosocial problems, PCTP did produce a reduction in psychosocial problems in children but had no statistically significant advantage over UC McCormick et al. (2014) Pediatric residents trained in Primary Care Triple P from 3 community clinics improved their parenting consultation skills and parents visiting these residents increased positive disciplinary strategies compared to parents visiting control residents. There were no differences found for child behavior or parenting sense of confidence Turner, Nicholson, and Sanders (2011) examined factors affecting the implementation by primary care practitioners (nursing, education, allied health, and medical) of Primary Care Triple P. Lack of compatibility at the program and workplace level (e.g., lack of clients, not appropriate for clients, limitations of normal work hours, lack of supervision) and difficulty of implementation (e.g., difficulties with time management, engaging clients, setting goals) were barriers to implementation. Flexibility (e.g., ability to tailor to individual needs) and training/preparation factors (e.g., knowledge and skills in BFI and behavior change) supported implementation				

(continued)

Table 4.2 (continued)

Program name	Evidence-based findings	Evidence in primary care with children 0–5 years	Discipline/educational qualifications of the practitioners	Target population	Cost (training, materials, supervision costs, any data re: cost per child served)	Required elements of the program
Video Interaction Project (VIP)	VIP is a primary care-based intervention for children birth to 5; therefore, the research conducted on its effectiveness has been in a primary care setting (please see next column)	Mendelsohn et al. (2007) VIP was associated with improved parenting practices, increased teaching behaviors, and lower levels of parenting stress. Additionally, VIP children were more likely to have normal cognitive developmental and less likely to have developmental delays in a randomized controlled trial Mendelsohn et al. (2011) Comparison of VIP vs. control group revealed VIP lead to increased parent–child interactions. The greatest effects were on mothers with a ninth-grade or higher reading level Berkule et al. (2014) Comparison study of interventions VIP and Building Blocks (BB) vs. a control group indicated lower rates of moderate depression for VIP mothers than for BB or the control group. Rates of mild depression were lower for VIP mothers than the control group	No specific qualifications are listed on the intervention website or other evidence-based databases	Parents and children, beginning at birth	The price of the VIP program could not be obtained from the website (Video Interaction Project, 2015)	The core components of the VIP program: Videotaped parent–child interactions Guided questions (Open-ended questions to guide families' observations and reactions to their child) Pamphlet (written pamphlet regarding development and behavior) Learning material (developmentally stimulating, age-appropriate toy and/or book)

Table 4.3 Costs

The chart below is an attempt to compare program costs. The task of cost comparison was a challenging one because each program differs in the level of services provided, types of materials, and a variety of other factors. Additionally, it should be noted that the chart below does not include travel costs such as airfare, lodging, and per diem, since such expenses are location specific. For some programs, it may be more cost efficient to have trainers travel to the trainees, a service several programs offer. When selecting trainers to come on-site, the maximum number of trainees allowed to attend trainings differs based on the program. To take this variation into account, we used a standardized number of 20 trainees when calculating the cost of training materials. We also indicate when the program allows for more than 20 trainees; however, we do not include the price of additional training materials in the estimated training cost. Finally, several programs provided a range for the program cost, without any explanation of factors that would increase or decrease costs. In these instances, we provided the cost range provided by the program. Hence, for a more specific budget, readers are encouraged to identify organization needs, select 1–3 programs that meet those needs, and then contact the specific programs directly for an organization-specific budget. The chart below aims to serve as a starting point in budget development. Often, due to the varying aspects of the program, direct comparison was not possible.

Program name	Training	Manual	Exam/certification	Consultation	Obligations to the program	Estimated cost
Child–Parent Psychotherapy (CPP) Total = $10,300 to $28,300 for 20 trainees (The California Evidence-Based Clearinghouse for Child Welfare 2015a & National Registry of Evidence-based Programs & Practices, 2015a)	Trainings occur 3 times over a 1.5-year period Each of the 3 trainings, occur for 2–3 days = 6–9 of total training days OPTION 1: Training at specialized NCTSN site through the NCTSN Learning Collaborative Model = Free. Plus travel, lodging, and per diem to training location for each trainee OPTION 2: On-site training with a maximum of 30 trainees = $1500–$3000/day On-site program must pay for the travel expenses for the trainer(s)	General Training Manual $40 ea./ ($800 for 20 trainees) Don't Hit My Mommy! Manual $25 ea./($500 for 20 trainees) Total = $1300	N/A	Phone, email, or in-person consultation $150–$350 per hour (in addition to the bimonthly phone consultation included in training cost)	Participating organizations agree to collect metrics and other outcome data	*A maximum of 30 trainees are allowed to attend on-site trainings. Numbers below reflect the price of 20 trainees and their training materials* $1300 training materials $1500–$3000/day Trainings are 6–9 days over 1.5-year period = $9000–$27,000 **Total = $10,300 to $28,300 for 20 trainees**

(continued)

Table 4.3 (continued)

Program name	Training	Manual	Exam/certification	Consultation	Obligations to the program	Estimated cost
Circle Of Security (COS) Total = $1240 (Parent Training and DVD)/$24,800 for 20 trainees $2840 (Intensive Training)/$56,800 for 20 trainees (Circle of Security, 2015)	Parent Training & DVD = $1000 for 1 trainee to be trained (plus travel, lodging, and per diem to training location) Intensive 10 Day Training – $2100–2400 (plus travel, lodging, and per diem to training location)	$40	$200	The availability of/cost of consultation is unknown		*On-site training options were not indicated on the program's website* Parent Training and DVD $1000 for training $40 manual $200 exam **Total = $1240 for 1 trainee/$24,800 for 20 trainees** (Australia, Canada, Italy, New Zealand, Norway, Romania, and the United States) Intensive Training $2400 for training $40 manual $200 exam **Total = $2640 for 1 trainee/$56,800 for 20 trainees** (plus travel, lodging, and per diem to Australia, Canada, or New Mexico)

Program name	Training	Manual	Exam/certification	Consultation	Obligations to the program	Estimated cost
Healthy Steps Total = $12,100–$18,100 for 20 trainees (Healthy Steps, 2015)	Getting started package – $100 The Training Institute – $12,000–$18,000 (includes travel, per diem, materials, and follow-up assistance for three Healthy Steps training faculty for 3 days)	Cost of handouts included in training costs	N/A	Follow-up assistance is available and included in training costs	Participating organizations agree to collect metrics and other outcome data	*The program did not indicate if there is a maximum number of trainees allowed to attend on-site trainings. Numbers below reflect the price of 20 trainees and their training materials* **Total = $12,100–18,100 for 20 trainees**
Incredible Years Total = $5700–$9345 for 20 trainees (National Registry of Evidence-based Programs and Practices 2015b)	OPTION 1: Training held in Seattle, Washington $500/per trainee for 3-day training workshop $375/per trainee for 2-day training workshop (plus travel, lodging, and per diem to training location) OPTION 2: On-site training—$1650–2000/day for any of the following options: 3 days for parent group leader training 2 days for baby program group leader training Plus half-day or 1-day travel day fee (this is variable, depending on your location or length of time to travel to your site)—charges based on the trainer daily fee, per above	$1150–$1895 depending on series selected $20 The Incredible Years: A Troubleshooting Guide ea./($400 for 20 trainees) $30 Collaborating with Parents to Reduce Children's Behavior Problems books ea./($600 for 20 trainees) $20 Incredible Babies ea./($400 for 20 trainees) $20 Handouts ea./($400 for 20 trainees) $1595 for DVD set (for Child programs)	$450 Certification fee (includes 2 video reviews)	$150–$200/h Telephone consultation by trainer $200 Consultation day in Seattle $90/h Extra video reviews by trainer (beyond 2 tapes for certification fee) Not included in total	Unclear	*A maximum of 25 trainees are allowed to attend on-site trainings. Numbers below reflect the price of 20 trainees and their training materials* $400–$600 Training manuals $400 Training handouts $1150–$1895 depending on series selected $3300–$6000 for on-site training $450 certification **Total = $5700–$9345 for 20 trainees**

(continued)

Table 4.3 (continued)

Program name	Training	Manual	Exam/certification	Consultation	Obligations to the program	Estimated cost
Parent–Child Interaction Therapy (PCIT) Total = $5200 for 1 trainee/$104,000 for 20 trainees (University of Colorado Boulder Institute of Behavioral Science, 2015a)	$4000 per trainee, (plus travel, lodging, and per diem to training location)	Included in training costs	$200 per organization	$1000 per year, per trainee	Unclear	*On-site training options were not indicated on the program's website. It is unclear if the price changes if there are less than four therapists and an administrator. Numbers below reflect the price of 1 and 20 trainee(s) and training materials* $4000 per trainee $200 per organization $1000 consultation/year **Total = $5200 for 1 trainee/$104,000 for 20 trainees** (plus travel, lodging, and per diem to training location)
The Triple P – Primary Care Triple P Total = $23,555 for 20 trainees (University of Colorado Boulder Institute of Behavioral Science, 2015b)	Level 3 – Primary Care Triple P 1 day pre-accreditation 2 day on-site training for up to 20 trainees – $23,555 It is unclear if the on-site program pays for the travel expenses for trainer(s)	Included in training costs		Included in training costs	Unclear	*A maximum of 20 trainees are allowed to attend on-site trainings. Numbers below reflect the price of 20 trainees and their training materials* Level 3 Primary Care Triple P = $23,555 Total = Primary Care Triple P = **$23,555 for 20 trainees**

Program name	Training	Manual	Exam/ certification	Consultation	Obligations to the program	Estimated cost
Video Interaction Project (VIP) Total = Unable to estimate (Video Interaction Project, 2015)	The price of the VIP program could not be obtained from the website or evidence-based database	The price of the VIP program could not be obtained from the website or evidence-based database	The price of the VIP program could not be obtained from the website or evidence-based database	The price of the VIP program could not be obtained from the website or evidence-based database	The price of the VIP program could not be obtained from the website or evidence-based database	The price of the VIP program could not be obtained from the website or evidence-based database

References

Berkovits, M. D., O'Brien, K. A., Carter, C. G., & Eyberg, S. M. (2010). Early identification and intervention for behavior problems in primary care: A comparison of two abbreviated versions of parent-child interaction therapy. *Behavior Therapy, 41*(3), 375–387.

Berkule, S. B., Cates, C. B., Dreyer, B. P., Huberman, H. S., Arevalo, J., Burtchen, N., ... Mendelsohn, A. L. (2014). Reducing maternal depressive symptoms through promotion of parenting in pediatric primary care. *Clinical Pediatrics, 53*(5), 460–469.

Berwick, D. M., Nolan, T. W., & Whittington, J. (2008). The triple aim: Care, health, and cost. *Health Affairs (Project Hope), 27*(3), 759–769.

Boggs, S. R., Eyberg, S. M., Edwards, D. L., Rayfield, A., Jacobs, J., Bagner, D., & Hood, K. K. (2005). Outcomes of parent-child interaction therapy: A comparison of treatment completers and study dropouts one to three years later. *Child & Family Behavior Therapy, 26*(4), 1–22.

Boyle, C. L., Sanders, M. R., Lutzker, J. R., Prinz, R. J., Shapiro, C., & Whitaker, D. J. (2010). An analysis of training, generalization, and maintenance effects of primary care triple P for parents of preschool-aged children with disruptive behavior. *Child Psychiatry & Human Development, 41*(1), 114–131.

Briggs, R. D., Silver, E. J., Krug, L. M., Mason, Z. S., Schrag, R. D., Chinitz, S., & Racine, A. D. (2014). Healthy steps as a moderator: The impact of maternal trauma on child social-emotional development. *Clinical Practice in Pediatric Psychology, 2*(2), 166.

Cassidy, J., Woodhouse, S. S., Sherman, L. J., Stupica, B., & Lejuez, C. (2011). Enhancing infant attachment security: An examination of treatment efficacy and differential susceptibility. *Development and Psychopathology, 23*(01), 131–148.

Caughy, M. O., Huang, K., Miller, T., & Genevro, J. L. (2004). The effects of the healthy steps for young children program: Results from observations of parenting and child development. *Early Childhood Research Quarterly, 19*(4), 611–630.

Chaffin, M., Silovsky, J. F., Funderburk, B., Valle, L. A., Brestan, E. V., Balachova, T., ... Bonner, B. L. (2004). Parent-child interaction therapy with physically abusive parents: Efficacy for reducing future abuse reports. *Journal of Consulting and Clinical Psychology, 72*(3), 500.

Child Parent Psychotherapy. (2015). Retrieved April 5, 2015 from http://childtrauma.ucsf.edu/child-parent-psychotherapy-training

Circle of Security. (2015). Retrieved April 5, 2015, from http://circleofsecurity.net/

Dowell, K. A., & Ogles, B. M. (2010). The effects of parent participation on child psychotherapy outcome: A meta-analytic review. *Journal of Clinical Child & Adolescent Psychology, 39*(2), 151–162.

Hagan, J. F., Shaw, J. S., & Duncan, P. M. (2008). *Bright futures: Guidelines for health supervision of infants, children, and adolescents*. Elk Grove Village, IL: American Academy of Pediatrics.

Healthy Steps. (2015). Retrieved April 5, 2015, from www.healthysteps.org.

Hoffman, K. T., Marvin, R. S., Cooper, G., & Powell, B. (2006). Changing toddlers' and pre-schoolers' attachment classifications: The circle of security intervention. *Journal of Consulting and Clinical Psychology, 74*(6), 1017.

Johnston, B. D., Huebner, C. E., Tyll, L. T., Barlow, W. E., & Thompson, R. S. (2004). Expanding developmental and behavioral services for newborns in primary care: Effects on parental well-being, practice, and satisfaction. *American Journal of Preventive Medicine, 26*(4), 356–366.

Lavigne, J. V., Lebailly, S. A., Gouze, K. R., Cicchetti, C., Pochyly, J., Arend, R., ... Binns, H. J. (2008). Treating oppositional defiant disorder in primary care: A comparison of three models. *Journal of Pediatric Psychology, 33*(5), 449–461.

Lieberman, A. F., Ippen, C. G., & Van Horn, P. (2006). Child-parent psychotherapy: 6-month follow-up of a randomized controlled trial. *Journal of the American Academy of Child & Adolescent Psychiatry, 45*(8), 913–918.

Liebhaber, A., & Grossman, J. M. (2007). Physicians moving to mid-sized, single-specialty practices. *Tracking Report/Center for Studying Health System Change, 18*, 1–5.

Markie-Dadds, C., & Sanders, M. R. (2006). Self-directed triple P (positive parenting program) for mothers with children at-risk of developing conduct problems. *Behavioural and Cognitive Psychotherapy, 34*(03), 259–275.

McConnell, D., Breitkreuz, R., & Savage, A. (2012). Independent evaluation of the triple P positive parenting program in family support service settings. *Child & Family Social Work, 17*(1), 43–54.

McCormick, E., Kerns, S. E., McPhillips, H., Wright, J., Christakis, D. A., & Rivara, F. P. (2014). Training pediatric residents to provide parent education: A randomized controlled trial. *Academic Pediatrics, 14*(4), 353–360.

McMenamy, J., Sheldrick, C., & Perrin, E. (2011). Early intervention in pediatrics offices for emerging disruptive behavior in toddlers. *Journal of Pediatric Health Care, 25*(2), 77–86.

Mendelsohn, A. L., Dreyer, B. P., Flynn, V., Tomopoulos, S., Rovira, I., Tineo, W., ... Nixon, A. F. (2005). Use of videotaped interactions during pediatric well-child care to promote child development: A randomized, controlled trial. *Journal of Developmental and Behavioral Pediatrics, 26*(1), 34–41.

Mendelsohn, A. L., Huberman, H. S., Berkule, S. B., Brockmeyer, C. A., Morrow, L. M., & Dreyer, B. P. (2011). Primary care strategies for promoting parent-child interactions and school readiness in at-risk families: The Bellevue project for early language, literacy, and education success. *Archives of Pediatrics & Adolescent Medicine, 165*(1), 33–41.

Mendelsohn, A. L., Valdez, P. T., Flynn, V., Foley, G. M., Berkule, S. B., Tomopoulos, S., ... Dreyer, B. P. (2007). Use of videotaped interactions during pediatric well-child care: Impact at 33 months on parenting and on child development. *Journal of Developmental and Behavioral Pediatrics, 28*(3), 206–212.

Minkovitz, C. S., Hughart, N., Strobino, D., Scharfstein, D., Grason, H., Hou, W., ... McLearn, K. T. (2003). A practice-based intervention to enhance quality of care in the first 3 years of life: The Healthy Steps for Young Children program. *JAMA, 290*(23), 3081–3091.

Minkovitz, C. S., Strobino, D., Mistry, K. B., Scharfstein, D. O., Grason, H., Hou, W., ... Guyer, B. (2007). Healthy Steps for Young Children: Sustained results at 5.5 years. *Pediatrics, 120*(3), e658–68.

Morawska, A., & Sanders, M. R. (2006). Self-administered behavioral family intervention for parents of toddlers: Part I. Efficacy. *Journal of Consulting and Clinical Psychology, 74*(1), 10.

National Registry of Evidence-based Programs and Practices. (2015a). *Child-Parent Psychotherapy (CPP)*. Retrieved November 29, 2015, from http://legacy.nreppadmin.net/ViewIntervention.aspx?id=194

National Registry of Evidence-based Programs and Practices. (2015b). *Incredible Years*. Retrieved November 29, 2015, from http://legacy.nreppadmin.net/ViewIntervention.aspx?id=311

National Registry of Evidence-based Programs and Practices. (2015c). *Parent-Child Interaction Therapy*. Retrieved November 29, 2015, fromhttp://legacy.nreppadmin.net/ViewIntervention.aspx?id=23

Nixon, R. D. (2001). Changes in hyperactivity and temperament in behaviourally disturbed vpreschoolers after parent–child interaction therapy (PCIT). *Behaviour Change, 18*(03), 168–176.

Parent Child Interaction Therapy (PCIT). (2015). Retrieved April 4, 2015, from http://www.pcit.org/

Perrin, E. C., Sheldrick, R. C., McMenamy, J. M., Henson, B. S., & Carter, A. S. (2014). Improving parenting skills for families of young children in pediatric settings: A randomized clinical trial. *JAMA Pediatrics, 168*(1), 16–24.

Piotrowski, C. C., Talavera, G. A., & Mayer, J. A. (2009). Healthy steps: A systematic review of a preventive practice-based model of pediatric care. *Journal of Developmental and Behavioral Pediatrics, 30*(1), 91–103.

Reedtz, C., Handegard, B. H., & Morch, W. (2011). Promoting positive parenting practices in primary care: Outcomes and mechanisms of change in a randomized controlled risk reduction trial. *Scandinavian Journal of Psychology, 52*(2), 131–137.

Sanders, M. R., Kirby, J. N., Tellegen, C. L., & Day, J. J. (2014). The triple P-positive parenting program: A systematic review and meta-analysis of a multi-level system of parenting support. *Clinical Psychology Review, 34*(4), 337–357.

Schappin, R., Wijnroks, L., Venema, M. U., Wijnberg-Williams, B., Veenstra, R., Koopman-Esseboom, C., ... Jongmans, M. (2014). Primary care triple P for parents of NICU graduates with behavioral problems: A randomized, clinical trial using observations of parent–child interaction. *BMC Pediatrics, 14*(1), 305.

Schuhmann, E. M., Foote, R. C., Eyberg, S. M., Boggs, S. R., & Algina, J. (1998). Efficacy of parent-child interaction therapy: Interim report of a randomized trial with short-term maintenance. *Journal of Clinical Child Psychology, 27*(1), 34–45.

Spijkers, W., Jansen, D. E., & Reijneveld, S. A. (2013). Effectiveness of primary care Triple P on child psychosocial problems in preventive child healthcare: A randomized controlled trial. *BMC Medicine, 11*, 240. doi: 10.1186/1741-7015-11-240.

The California Evidence-Based Clearinghouse for Child Welfare. (2015a). *Child-Parent Psychotherapy (CPP)*. Retrieved April 4, 2015, from http://www.cebc4cw.org/program/child-parent-psychotherapy/detailed

The California Evidence-Based Clearinghouse for Child Welfare. (2015b). *Circle of Security Parenting*. (2015). Retrieved from April 4, 2015, from http://www.cebc4cw.org/program/circle-of-security-parenting/detailed

The Incredible Years. (2015). Retrieved April 4, 2015, from http://www.incredibleyears.com

Toth, S. L., Maughan, A., Manly, J. T., Spagnola, M., & Cicchetti, D. (2002). The relative efficacy of two interventions in altering maltreated preschool children's representational models: Implications for attachment theory. *Development and Psychopathology, 14*(04), 877–908.

Toth, S. L., Rogosch, F. A., Manly, J. T., & Cicchetti, D. (2006). The efficacy of toddler-parent psychotherapy to reorganize attachment in the young offspring of mothers with major depressive disorder: A randomized preventive trial. *Journal of Consulting and Clinical Psychology, 74*(6), 1006.

Triple P Parenting. (2015). Retrieved April 4, 2015, from http://www.triplep.net/glo-en/home/

Turner, K. M., Nicholson, J. M., & Sanders, M. R. (2011). The role of practitioner self-efficacy, training, program and workplace factors on the implementation of an evidence-based parenting intervention in primary care. *The Journal of Primary Prevention, 32*(2), 95–112.

Turner, K. M., & Sanders, M. R. (2006). Help when it's needed first: A controlled evaluation of brief, preventive behavioral family intervention in a primary care setting. *Behavior Therapy, 37*(2), 131–142.

University of Colorado Boulder Institute of Behavioral Science. (2015a). *Parent-child interaction therapy (PCIT)*. Retrieved April 5, 2015, from http://www.blueprintsprograms.com/factSheet.php?pid=50336bc687eb161ee9fb0ddb8cf2b7e65bad865f

University of Colorado Boulder Institute of Behavioral Science. (2015b). *Blueprints for healthy youth development: Triple P system program cost*. Retrieved April 4, 2015, from http://www.blueprintsprograms.com/factSheet.php?pid=07fd89a40a3755e21a5884640f23eaf59b66df35

Video Interaction Project (VIP). (2015). Retrieved April 5, 2015, from http://childrenofbellevue.org/video-interaction-project/

Webster-Stratton, C. H., Reid, M. J., & Beauchaine, T. (2011). Combining parent and child training for young children with ADHD. *Journal of Clinical Child & Adolescent Psychology, 40*(2), 191–203.

Chapter 5
Healthy Steps for Young Children: Integrating Behavioral Health into Primary Care for Young Children and their Families

Margot Kaplan-Sanoff and Rahil D. Briggs

Abstract Pediatric clinicians have been tasked by the American Academy of Pediatrics with increasing their attention to the psychosocial determinants of health for early childhood, including the prevention and treatment of toxic stress. To help practices as they struggle to design a comprehensive response to this call, this chapter presents the Healthy Steps program, a flexible model of integrated primary pediatric care that has been adapting to change in healthcare and reimbursement practices and policies since its inception in 1994. Currently operating in over 80 sites nationwide, Healthy Steps expands the model of a solo pediatric clinician to include a new member of the healthcare team—the Healthy Steps Specialist—who enhances the information and services available to parents by providing specific information about the child's behavior and development, by discussing the family's adjustment to caring for their new baby, and by conducting screening and intervention related to the additional psychosocial needs of the child and/or family.

Keywords Healthy Steps • Pediatric care • Behavioral health

> "Just when I thought I had my 4 month old on a sleep schedule, he started waking up several times in the middle of the night."

> "I was so proud of myself and bragging to my friends that my little girl enjoyed eating everything, even vegetables. Then all of a sudden she started saying "No!" and refused to eat anything but fruits."

Change, and adjusting to change, is a constant reality in the lives of parents raising infants and toddlers. Change, too, is becoming the new normal for healthcare practices as updated information on genetics, brain development, and the impact of trauma on young children becomes available and insurance practices/policies/eligi-

M. Kaplan-Sanoff, Ed.D. (✉)
Healthy Steps, Zero to Three, Washington, DC, USA
e-mail: msanoff@gmail.com

R.D. Briggs, Psy.D.
Montefiore Health System, Bronx, NY, USA
e-mail: rabriggs@montefiore.org

© Springer International Publishing Switzerland 2016
R.D. Briggs (ed.), *Integrated Early Childhood Behavioral Health in Primary Care*, DOI 10.1007/978-3-319-31815-8_5

bility are endlessly revised (Coker, Chung, Cowgill, Chen, & Rodriguez, 2009). As per the American Academy of Pediatrics (Garner, Shonkoff, Committee on Psychosocial Aspects of Child and Family Health, Early Childhood, Adoption, Dependent, and Section on Developmental and Behavioral Pediatrics 2012), pediatric practice have been tasked with increasing their attention to the psychosocial determinants of health for early childhood, including the prevention and treatment of toxic stress. As practices struggle to design a comprehensive response to this call, in this chapter we present the Healthy Steps program, a flexible model of integrated primary pediatric care that has been adapting to change since its inception in 1994.

Healthy Steps for Young Children

Healthy Steps was launched by Ms. Margaret Mahoney, then Executive Director of The Commonwealth Fund, and cosponsored by the American Academy of Pediatrics. The Fund's goals were to:

- apply new scientific discoveries regarding child behavior and development to medical practices,
- design and test a new approach to primary care for young children that would provide mothers and fathers and clinicians with information and support,
- inform mothers and fathers, business leaders, public officials, and healthcare professionals about the importance of the first 3 years of life.

A small team of developmental pediatricians, pediatric nurse practitioners, and child development specialists at Boston University School of Medicine was chosen to develop the model and design the training curriculum for Healthy Steps. What resulted is a national initiative that emphasizes a close relationship between healthcare professionals and parents in addressing the physical, emotional, and intellectual growth and development of children from birth to age three (McLearn, Zuckerman, Parker, Yelowitz, & Kaplan-Sanoff, 1998). In a traditional pediatric practice, one pediatric clinician typically tries to address all of the child's health and developmental needs. Healthy Steps expands the model of a solo pediatric clinician to include a new member of the healthcare team—the Healthy Steps Specialist— who enhances the information and services available to parents by providing specific information about the child's behavior and development, by discussing the family's adjustment to caring for this baby, and by conducting screening to determine additional psychosocial needs of the child and/or family.

The Healthy Steps Specialist (HSS) can be a new team member or a nurse, child development specialist, or early childhood behavioral health clinician already working in the practice. Healthy Steps Specialists have specialized training in child development, early intervention, early childhood behavioral health, counseling, or nursing and can address major behavioral and developmental issues, focusing on the child within the context of the family. Many Healthy Steps Specialists have additional training in infant mental health and trauma informed care. The Healthy

Steps Specialist is the primary child development and family support resource for families, bringing to the practice an expertise in child and family development (Kaplan-Sanoff, Lerner, & Bernard, 2000). Healthy Steps Specialists comanage families with pediatric clinicians, ensuring that the practice has the time and expertise to address each family's need for information and support.

The cornerstone of all Healthy Steps programs is relationship-based practice which includes:

1. Building relationships as a primary goal of providing services to children and families,
2. Recognizing that the relationship between parents and the clinician is fundamental to quality services,
3. Focusing on promoting the parent–child relationship,
4. Emphasizing that all behavior has meaning, even a young infant's cry or a toddler's refusal to eat.

Healthy Steps helps parents consider their child's behavior in the context of the child's intended meaning. They might ask questions such as "What do you think the baby is trying to tell you when she throws her food off the high chair?" or "What's your understanding about why your mother wants you to discipline your child for touching her breakables?" Relationship-based practice highlights the parents' expertise and asks for their hunch as to what the child's behavior might mean; it promotes perspective-taking and conveys the notion of reciprocity between all parties that the Healthy Steps team and the family will figure this out together.

Healthy Steps practices accomplish the goal of providing relationship-based practice by using a team approach, allowing both the pediatric clinician and the Healthy Steps Specialist to interact together in the same exam room with the family when they come in for well-child visits (Zuckerman, Kaplan-Sanoff, Parker, & Young, 1997). As a team, they build on each other's knowledge and resources, responding to parental questions and concerns with both a medical focus and a behavioral/developmental perspective (Kaplan-Sanoff, M. 2013). For example, when a family voices concern about their child's eating, the pediatric clinician might use the growth chart to reassure the family about the baby's weight gain. Then the Healthy Steps Specialist might ask about the family's routines for feeding, their expectations about the baby's eating, and whether this concern is based on feedback from other family members or friends.

This team approach to primary care offers families enhanced well-child visits which emphasize the promotion of children's development, including strategies to improve the "goodness of fit" between parent and child, closer attention to parental questions and concerns, and the use of "teachable moments" to support better parental understanding of their child's behavior, and support for early literacy (Zuckerman, Parker, Kaplan-Sanoff, Augustyn, & Barth, 2004). An enhanced Healthy Steps visit may be conducted jointly or sequentially by the pediatric clinician and Healthy Steps Specialist.

Other critical components of Healthy Steps include:

- Home visits by the HSS, timed to specific developmental needs in young children,
- A dedicated child development telephone or text messaging information line,
- Child development and "family health checkups," including developmental screening for the children and risk and protective factor screening for the parents,
- Tighter linkages and facilitated referrals to community resources,
- Written materials for parents that emphasize prevention and health promotion within the context of their relationships with family,
- Pediatric and community resources, and parent support groups.

In 1998, the Johns Hopkins Bloomberg School of Public Health rigorously evaluated Healthy Steps using medical record review, parent and provider satisfaction and knowledge questionnaires, telephone interviews, and contact logs. Initial 3-year data reported in JAMA indicate that for all children, not just those at high risk, the quality of pediatric care in the first 3 years of life was dramatically improved due to Healthy Steps; by changing the structure and process of pediatric care, Healthy Steps significantly improved the delivery of pediatric developmental services (Minkovitz et al., 2003). The randomized controlled trial evaluation found that, among other results, families involved in the Healthy Steps program were more likely than non-participating families to:

- Discuss concerns with someone in the practice about a variety of issues such as the importance of routines, discipline, language development, child's temperament, and sleeping patterns,
- Demonstrate greater security of attachment and fewer behavior problems,
- Significantly increase the use of inductive forms of discipline and a subsequent reduction of harsh physical punishment,
- Be highly satisfied with care because someone in the practice went out of their way for them,
- Ensure that infants slept on their back to help reduce the risk of Sudden Infant Death Syndrome (SIDS),
- Receive timely well-child visits and vaccinations,
- Experience continuity of care with parents choosing to remain with the practice until the child was at least 20 months old.

Healthy Steps helped parents better understand their children's behavior and development, thereby producing more favorable disciplinary practices. Pediatric clinicians were highly satisfied with the program and viewed Healthy Steps as a valuable service that helped to keep families in their practices. Minkovitz and colleagues also conducted a 5-year follow-up study of Healthy Steps children and families (Minkovitz et al., 2007) and determined that the beneficial results from participating in Healthy Steps lasted for at least 2 years after the completion of the intervention. At that time parents continued to use less severe discipline, remained highly satisfied with their practice (in part because they received timely anticipatory guidance), and reported that their children spent more time looking at books.

Screening as a Vehicle for Parental Understanding of Child Development and Behavior

Developmental and social-emotional screening of children and screening parents for risk and protective factors have always been components of Healthy Steps. Screening can be conducted by the pediatric clinician (especially if the clinician is a resident and needs to learn how to screen effectively) or by the Healthy Steps Specialists in either an office well-child visit or during a home visit. Most HS practices are currently using the Ages and Stages Questionnaire-3 (ASQ-3; Squires & Bricker, 2009) and Ages and Stages Social-Emotional (ASQ:SE; Squires, Bricker, & Twombly, 2002) screeners, and the Modified Checklist for Autism in Toddlers-Revised (MCHAT-R; Robins, Fein, & Barton, 2009) at 15–18 months. In addition, Healthy Steps Specialists often complete a temperament scale with parents and their 4-month-olds to promote goodness of fit between families and their infants, to help parents better understand their expectations for their child and themselves, and to introduce a construct for helping parents predict and adjust to their child's temperamental characteristics when faced with new challenges, such as separation in child care, trying solid foods, toilet training, and sibling/peer relationships. Better understanding of their child's temperament and their own temperamental characteristics can help parents feel more confident in the child-rearing decisions they are making for their child.

Consideration of parental behavior/responses to their children is another aspect of the Healthy Steps two-generational model of care. Healthy Steps asks families to consider the risk and protective factors which they might bring to their parenting, as adult behaviors such as smoking, substance abuse, depression, anxiety, and intimate partner violence have been shown to be harmful to children, especially in the first 3 years of life. They are a clear risk to children's health and behavior and, in severe form, are considered adverse childhood experiences which later impact child health, mental health, and development (Felitti et al., 1998; Shonkoff et al., 2012). In addition, the birth of a baby is often a window of opportunity for parents to consider changes to their behavior. Parents want to do better for their infants and young children and, in the first few months after birth, they are very open to considering changes in their behavior. Children can be powerful motivators for parental change; many parents have already made significant changes to their behavior during the pregnancy by changing diet, drinking, or smoking habits. The success of Healthy Steps is supported by the relationship that exists between a child's parent(s), a pediatric clinician, and the Healthy Steps team, and the accessibility of the team for repeated contact with parents over time, allowing for follow-up and support. The very act of asking about adult risk factors and parental behavior by the Healthy Steps team offers parents the opportunity to consider concerns about their behavior, and identifies the HS team as a place where they can talk about their issues. Finally, Healthy Steps teams ask about parental behavior because there is a serious risk of under-identifying parental mental health issues which have the potential to be treated (Kaplan-Sanoff, M. 2006).

Risk factors are not automatically predictive of child behavior due to the presence of protective factors, such as community resources including Early Head Start, quality child care, home visiting, early intervention programs, pastoral counseling, and kin and kith care with adults who act as protective factors for the child and offer respite to the parents as they work on changing their behavior (Satcher, 2001). Additional protective factors, including parental resilience, knowledge of parenting and child development, social and emotional competence of children, social connections, and concrete supports are also considered as part of a well-child visit. For example, Healthy Steps teams ask families if they have enough food to feed their children for the coming week; based on the reply, Healthy Steps Specialists can follow up with a discussion of The Special Supplemental Nutrition Program for Women, Infants, and Children (WIC), Supplemental Nutrition Assistance Program (SNAP), and support for how to access a local food bank.

Healthy Steps routinely screens for:

- Exposure to smoking
- Maternal depression
- Alcohol/substance abuse
- Intimate partner violence
- Community violence
- Parents' childhood experiences, including Adverse Childhood Experiences (ACEs)
- Guns in the home
- Family incarceration
- Parental strengths/resilience
- Support systems: family, community
- Income Screening: Food insecurity, Transitional Aid to Families with Dependent Children (TAFDC), Supplemental Security Income (SSI)
- Housing and utilities screening: utility shut-off protection; housing stability; health concerns re: housing
- Education: child care vouchers; concerns about child's learning or behavior in school
- Employment
- Immigration status

For the Healthy Steps team, the screening process does not begin and end with conducting the screen. How the screening process is introduced, how parents understand their level of participation in the screening of their child, and how feedback is framed and delivered after the screen are as important as administering the screen. The screening process creates teachable moments, those times during the well-child visit when parents may be more open and receptive to discussion about their child's behavior/development and other family stress. To help the Healthy Steps team provide effective information and support for parents within the time constraints of a typical office visit, the use of Teachable Moments (TM) represents a highly effective strategy (Parker & Zuckerman, 2004). By using the basic assessments of the pediatric visit—history taking, physical examinations, and developmental screening—as potential teachable moments, the team can exploit the educational opportunities they present for intervention. The strategy of teachable moments is to use the behavior of the child during the screening process and the adult-child interactions observed in the office, as shared experiences that further parents' insights into their child and enhance their sense of competence as parents. The goals of teachable moments are to:

- Enhance parents' understanding of the child's needs,
- Promote "goodness of fit" between parent and child,
- Model constructive interactions with the child,
- Enhance the relationship between the Healthy Steps team and the parent.

The developmental checkup creates the perfect teachable moment to form or enhance a supportive alliance between the Healthy Steps team and the family by addressing parents as individuals in their own right and adopting a collaborative stance when sharing observations about the child's behavior during the screening process. The team promotes goodness of fit by helping the parents understand their child's temperament, and, via an understanding of their own temperamental characteristics, parents clarify their expectations, aspirations, and caregiving style. For example, highlighting the child's persistence at a task as a positive learning style can help the parent reframe their interpretation of the child as "stubborn," and "she never gives in." Using the screening as an opportunity to enhance the parent's understanding of their child makes screening a welcomed, collaborative process, as both the Healthy Steps team and the parents observe the child's attempts to complete tasks. It can also set the stage for anticipatory guidance as new skills begin to emerge. A focus on the strengths of the child and family can put problems into context and modify the pathological model so stressful for parents of young children. To ensure that parents leave with a clear understanding of the screening results and the possible next steps, the team asks parents indirectly what they have understood about the process by personalizing the question. For example, "I know that his father is anxious to hear what we discovered today during the visit, what will you tell him?" This simple question allows the team to address both the child and family's strengths and concerns and to determine if the family has understood the implications of the screening results and next steps for their child.

Changes and Adaptations to Healthy Steps

Healthy Steps now operates in many diverse pediatric and family medicine sites (in 2015, over 500 pediatric clinicians, family physicians, and pediatric and family medicine residents are participating in Healthy Steps). With the recent availability of federal funding streams such as Project LAUNCH from the Substance Abuse and Mental Health Services Administration (SAMHSA) and the Affordable Care Act Maternal Infant Early Childhood Home Visiting (ACA MIECHV) which has funded new Healthy Steps sites, there have been some creative adaptations to the implementation of the model. In several communities, public health agencies and early care and education programs have also been awarded grants to collaborate with pediatric and family medicine practices to implement Healthy Steps using staff from the community agency to work in the practices. With the potential of additional funding for services provided by Healthy Steps to sites certified as Patient Centered Medical Homes, there is considerable interest in implementing Healthy Steps. The current diversity of Healthy Steps sites includes:

- Academic Health Centers
- Community Health Centers
- Private practices
- Hospital-based clinics
- Family Medicine practices
- Federally Qualified Health Centers
- Patient Centered Medical Homes
- NICU follow-up
- Residency Training Programs
  - Hospital-based training programs
  - Residency training rotations sites

Many of the newer sites coming on board have been family practice sites and have been very interested in providing a prenatal component for Healthy Steps, as they can track their prenatal patients who will continue to have their infants seen in primary care. The National HS Office currently offers a three visit prenatal home visiting component for families who are enrolled prenatally in Healthy Steps. This provides even greater continuity of care for families and insures better follow-up postpartum for mothers and babies. Finally, many Healthy Steps sites have trained their Healthy Steps Specialist to be lactation consultants, available to mothers who have questions or concerns in this area.

Infusing Fussy Baby into Healthy Steps

In 2013–2014, all Healthy Steps Specialists were invited to participate in FAN (Facilitating Attuned Interaction) training provided by the Fussy Baby Network® team at Erikson Institute (Gilkerson et al., 2012; Gilkerson & Gray, 2014). The FAN is a conceptual model and practical tool for attunement in relationships and for reflective practice. The FAN Core Processes are:

- Empathic Inquiry to support parents around feelings,
- Collaborative Exploration to think together with parents about their concerns,
- Capacity Building to increase parents' confidence and competence in caring for their child,
- Integration, to validate parents' insights on their child and their parenting,
- Mindful Self-Regulation.

Using this fifth core process, Healthy Steps Specialists are able to notice and regulate their own emotional responses in challenging moments in interactions and then engage with calm awareness in the interaction.

FAN also offers Healthy Steps Specialists a way to slow down and structure their interactions with families using the FAN Arc of Engagement questions: at the beginning of the visit, asking for the parents' experience ("How has it been going for YOU caring for your child?"); checking in at the middle to make the visit more family-led ("Are we getting to what you most wanted to talk about?"); and at the end, asking parents to reflect on their child by describing him/her in three words and asking what the parent would like to remember or carry with them from the visit.

With funding from the Doris Duke Charitable Foundation, we were able to offer three regional trainings in Florida, Illinois and Arizona to train Healthy Steps Specialists to infuse the principles and strategies of the FAN into their Healthy Steps practice, thereby giving them additional tools to work with families struggling with infant crying, sleep, irritability, and other common behavioral or developmental challenges. The Healthy Steps Specialists found this an extremely effective and viable way to engage with families. Specialists reported positive changes using the FAN; for example in one site, the parents were more up-to-date on their well-child checks, parents remembered and used the resource line more, and there was more engagement with young parents in the actual visits. Using the ARC of Engagement questions, the Specialists reported they had more "face-to-face time" with teen parents who had been disengaged on their phones and looking away. Now, the parents were more attentive and involved, expecting to be asked how it was going for them as a parent and knowing the visit would be focused on their concerns. Other Healthy Steps Specialists found the approach helpful in communication with care team members, using Mindful Self-Regulation to stay calm during difficult interactions and stressful moments in a busy practice.

In addition, several sites identified the need for in-house mental health services for families who were struggling with the trauma of poverty, homelessness, isolation, domestic violence, and immigration (Kaplan-Sanoff, Talmi, & Augustyn, 2013). These sites such as Montefiore Medical Group in the Bronx, NY employ licensed mental health clinicians, usually licensed psychologists, as Healthy Steps Specialists. These HSS provide mental health services to families within the context of the non-stigmatizing environment of a pediatric visit (Briggs, Germán, & Schrag, 2013). Please see more about the Montefiore model in Chap. 7 of this volume.

Implementing Healthy Steps in the Real World: Lessons Learned from the Sites

Instituting any change in a complex system requires planning and careful consideration of the potential pitfalls of enacting that change. Experienced Healthy Steps sites offer the following suggestions:

1. Identify a champion, usually a pediatric clinician, who has the power to make change in the organization and can "rally the troops" to join in implementation.
2. Set a "big table" and invite everyone in the practice to participate in decision-making that impacts their work whenever possible. Include the nurses,

PAs, receptionists, back-office staff, etc., in an orientation about Healthy Steps. Discuss how it may change their job responsibilities, including the need to schedule both the pediatric clinician and the HSS for well-child visits with Healthy Steps families.

3. Acknowledge the work that came before to avoid resentment. Other staff may have worked hard to insure continuity of care for new families and should be recognized for that effort.

4. Plan training opportunities so that all staff have the opportunity to discuss the ideas and changes being implemented. Remember that "all politics is local" and get a lay of the land including perceived competition in the community, governmental supports and regulations, barriers to care, and other "deal killers." The more you know about potential roadblocks to change, the better you can anticipate possible resistance to implementing a model of care that integrates behavioral health into primary care for young children and their families.

5. Articulate clear messages to families about what they can expect from Healthy Steps.

6. Articulate clear outcomes for pediatric clinicians and staff so they know what they can expect.

7. Expect and acknowledge unintended outcomes. Many sites were surprised that Healthy Steps families were more assertive in making their needs and concerns known to the support staff.

8. Celebrate small changes with the entire practice.

9. Balance requirements with flexibility so that support staff don't feel like implementing Healthy Steps is just another task, rather than a positive change for the practice and for the families.

Challenges

The Healthy Steps sites that have been operating over the past 20 years have also highlighted the challenges that arise when a medical practice focuses on relationship-based care. Pediatric clinicians worry about "opening a can of worms" when asking families for their ideas on why a child might be behaving in a concerning way; they worry about the time it will take to explore an issue with a family; and they worry about interfering with office flow when they know the waiting room is packed. While these are certainly valid concerns, having a Healthy Steps Specialist share the visit means that the Specialist can continue the discussion with the family, either in the exam room or in another office where the family can feel comfortable discussing their worries. The Specialist can also offer a home visit or a follow-up phone call to continue to work with the family. And while it may take a few weeks for the practice to adjust to the scheduling requirements of Healthy Steps, all practices report that after an initial period of adjustment Healthy Steps does not significantly interrupt office flow. In addition, parents report being more satisfied with their visits, because while they are waiting for the pediatric clinician, they are engaged in conversation with the Healthy Steps Specialist. A second challenge often voiced by pediatricians is related to the documentation of parental mental health concerns in the child's medical record, while recognizing confidentiality concerns. This is especially true when the adult risk screening identifies a family member who might need additional help with depression, substance abuse, or domestic violence. Please see Chap. 7 of this volume for more discussion of this matter.

Healthy Steps 2015 and Beyond: Future Changes

The National Office of Healthy Steps recently transferred from the Boston University School of Medicine to ZERO TO THREE. ZERO TO THREE is the preeminent national organization whose mission is to promote the health and development of infants and toddlers (www.zerotothree.org). ZERO TO THREE has focused for more than 30 years on the needs of infants, toddlers, and their families. The organization's unique resources offer expanded materials and training opportunities to support, sustain, and enhance the community of learning among all Healthy Steps sites and to offer new opportunities for professional development. Resources include the recently launched Parenting Portal that contains a collection of videos, podcasts, and downloadable resources for parents and professionals who work with parents. The portal can be accessed at http://www.zerotothree.org/parenting-resources/.

ZERO TO THREE has secured funding to examine effective replication, sustainability, and scalability pathways for the Healthy Steps model. The goal is to build the capacity and infrastructure of the National Healthy Steps Office at ZERO TO THREE to design a blueprint for the next stage of growth and evaluation. The funding has allowed the National Office to hire a Director of Finance and Sustainability who will work with state Medicaid offices and other public and private entities to determine appropriate funding streams to sustain Healthy Steps programs through billing and reimbursement strategies. Funding will also allow the National Office to collaborate with an evaluation firm to codify the program model and develop clearly defined fidelity and outcome indicators. In addition, the National Office will create a scaling study to develop a road map for a large-scale implementation by assessing market conditions, the competitive landscape, and funding pathways. This will include the development of a multiyear implementation plan with key activities/strategies required to successfully execute the growth of Healthy Steps.

With change comes growth and risk. Working closely with the existing Healthy Steps sites and experts in the field of implementation and sustainability, the National Office hopes to minimize risks for individual sites while enhancing the growth potential for expansion at existing and new sites across the country. There are currently over 80 Healthy Steps sites up and running, and we look forward to continued growth.

References

Briggs, R. D., Germán, M., & Schrag, R. D. A. (2013). Breaking down silos with a butter knife: Lessons learned from integrated pediatric behavioral health. *New York State Psychologist, 25*(4), 31–34.

Coker, T. R., Chung, P. J., Cowgill, B. O., Chen, L., & Rodriguez, M. A. (2009). Low-income parents' views on the redesign of well-child care. *Pediatrics, 124*(1), 194–204.

Felitti, V. J., Anda, R. F, Nordenberg, D., Williamson, D. F, Spitz, A. M., Edwards, V., … Marks, J. S. (1998). Relationship of childhood abuse and household dysfunction to many of the leading causes of death in adults: The Adverse Childhood Experiences (ACE) Study. *American Journal of Preventive Medicine, 14*:245–258.

Garner, A. S., & Shonkoff, J. P., Committee on Psychosocial Aspects of Child and Family Health, Committee on Early Childhood, Adoption, and Dependent Care, Section on Developmental and Behavioral Pediatrics. (2012). Early childhood adversity, toxic stress, and the role of the pediatrician: translating developmental science into lifelong health. *Pediatrics, 129*(1). Retrieved from www.pediatrics.org/cgi/content/full/129/1/e224

Gilkerson, L., & Gray, L. (2014). Fussy babies: Early challenges in regulation, impact on the dyad and family, and longer-term implications. In K. Brandt, B. Perry, S. Seligman, & E. Tronick (Eds.), *Infant and early childhood mental health* (pp. 195–208). Alexandria, VA: American Psychiatric.

Gilkerson, L, Hofherr, J., Steir, A., Cook, A., Arbel, A., Heffron, M., … Paul, J. (2012) Implementing fussy baby network approach. *Zero to Three Journal, 33*(2), 59–65.

Kaplan-Sanoff, M. (2006). Infusing mental health support and services into pediatric primary care. In D. F. Perry, R. K. Kaufmann, & J. Knitzer (Eds.), *Social and emotional health in early childhood*. Baltimore, MD: Brookes.

Kaplan-Sanoff, M. (2013). Healthy Steps for Young Children: Supporting young children and their families using primary care as a vehicle for service delivery. In "North American Models." In Glascoe FP, Marks KP, Poon JK, Macias MM (Eds.). Identifying and Addressing Developmental-Behavioral Problems: A Practical Guide for Medical and Non-medical Professionals, Trainees, Researchers and Advocates. Nolensville, TN: PEDSTest.com, LLC

Kaplan-Sanoff, M., Lerner, C., & Bernard, A. (2000). New roles for developmental specialists in pediatric primary care. *Zero to Three, 18*(2), 17–23.

Kaplan-Sanoff, M., Talmi, A., & Augustyn, M. (2013). Infusing mental health services into primary care for very young children and their families. *Zero-to-Three Journal, 33*(2), 73–77.

McLearn, K., Zuckerman, B., Parker, S., Yelowitz, M., & Kaplan-Sanoff, M. (1998). Child development and pediatrics for the 21st century: The healthy steps approach. *Journal of Urban Health, 75*(4), 704–723.

Minkovitz, C.S., Hughart, N., Strobin, D., Scharfstein, D., Grason, H., Hou, M., … Guyer, B. (2003) A practice-based intervention to enhance quality of care in the first three years of life: Results from the healthy steps for young children program. *Journal of the American Medical Association, 290*(23), 3081–3091.

Minkovitz, C. S., Strobino, D., Mistry, K. B., Scharfstein, D. O., Grason, H., Hou, W., & Guyer, B. (2007). Healthy steps for young children: Sustained results at 5.5 years. *Pediatrics, 120*(3), 658–668.

Parker, S., & Zuckerman, B. (2004). Teachable moments in primary care. In S. Parker, B. Zuckerman, & M. Augustyn (Eds.), *Handbook of developmental and behavioral pediatrics: A handbook for primary care* (2nd ed.). Boston, MA: Lippincott, Williams & Wilkins.

Robins, D. L., Fein, D., & Barton, M. (2009). The modified checklist for autism in toddlers. Revised (M-CHAT-R). Self-published.

Satcher, D. (2001). Surgeon General's Report on Youth Violence. US Dept of Health and Human Services Office of the Surgeon General, Public Health Service, United States of America.

Shonkoff, J. P., Garner, A. S., Committee on Psychosocial Aspects of Child and Family Health, Committee on Early Childhood, Adoption, and Dependent Care, & Section on Developmental and Behavioral Pediatrics. (2012). The lifelong effects of early childhood adversity and toxic stress. *Pediatrics, 129*(1), e232–e246.

Squires, J., & Bricker, D. (2009). *Ages and stages questionnaires, third edition (ASQ-3)*. Baltimore, MD: Paul H. Brookes.

Squires, J., Bricker, D., & Twombly, E. (2002). *Ages and stages questionnaire: Social-emotional (ASQ:SE)*. Baltimore, MD: Paul H. Brookes.

Zuckerman, B., Kaplan-Sanoff, M., Parker, S., & Young, K. (1997). The healthy steps for young children program. *Zero-to-Three, 17*(6), 20–25.

Zuckerman, B., Parker, S., Kaplan-Sanoff, M., Augustyn, A., & Barth, M. (2004). Healthy steps: A case study of innovation in pediatric practice. *Pediatrics, 114*(3), 820–826.

Chapter 6
Workforce Development for Integrated Early Childhood Behavioral Health

Rebecca Schrag Hershberg and Rahil D. Briggs

Abstract When looking to implement an early childhood integrated behavioral health program, it is critical to consider issues related to workforce development. In this chapter, we outline the suggested areas of knowledge and particular skill sets necessary for early childhood integrated behavior health specialists to be effective in this role. We also raise questions primary care pediatric practices need to address when determining who best to fill this position, particular to their type and scope of service. Practical examples are used to illustrate important topics, and strategies for incorporating ongoing interdisciplinary training are discussed.

Keywords Early childhood • Behavioral health • Integrated care • Workforce development • Interdisciplinary training

Introduction

When considering workforce development in early childhood integrated behavioral health, there are two critical parts of the equation: the work and the force. In other words, there are two questions to ask. First, what are the tasks and requirements of the job, the unique skills and abilities that are needed to do the work most effectively? Second, who are the best people to fill the positions, and what qualities and traits do they need in order to function successfully? And finally, once those two questions have been adequately addressed, what is the "development" piece to ensure continual training and ongoing effectiveness?

It is also important to note that workforce development is not only about training individuals to serve as integrated early childhood behavioral health specialists, but also about helping a primary care practice to evolve, and to be open to what is, essentially, a culture change. So, for example, implementing trainings for pediatricians, working with nursing and front desk staff to create screening work flows—all of this is a part of developing a workforce that functions capably and collaboratively within an integrated care setting.

R.S. Hershberg, Ph.D. (✉) • R.D. Briggs, Psy.D.
Montefiore Health System, Bronx, NY, USA
e-mail: drschrag@littlehousecalls.com; rabriggs@montefiore.org

© Springer International Publishing Switzerland 2016
R.D. Briggs (ed.), *Integrated Early Childhood Behavioral Health in Primary Care*, DOI 10.1007/978-3-319-31815-8_6

The "Work" in Workforce

There is no one career path that lends itself exclusively to becoming an integrated early childhood behavioral health practitioner. As reviewed in Chap. 4 by Crawford and Briggs in this volume, a review of the literature on evidence-based integrated early childhood behavioral health programs revealed that these practitioners may span a range of professional backgrounds and credentials. The most common are mental health professionals of all levels (M.A., S.W., Ph.D.), early childhood educators, nurses, and paraprofessionals.

Due to this heterogeneity, rather than attempt to define the "unique role" of an early childhood integrated behavioral health specialist, we believe it will be most useful to expound upon the areas of knowledge and particular skill sets needed to be able to do this work in the most effective manner. The following is our proposed "checklist" of what successful early childhood integrated behavioral health specialists need to know at a minimum.

Normal Early Childhood Development

As one of the primary functions of these practitioners is to provide guidance to parents about the developmental trajectories of their infants and toddlers, an extensive knowledge and understanding of normal childhood development is essential. Early childhood integrated behavioral health specialists need to know all of the milestones—across all major domains (cognitive, gross and fine motor, language, behavior, social–emotional)—that characterize typical infant and toddler development, as well as strategies for optimizing the likelihood that these milestones will occur along the expected and desired timeline. Such knowledge is critical not only to provide appropriate anticipatory guidance to parents, but also to be able to model and teach ways to encourage young children's growth in myriad and creative ways. Moreover, practitioners need to be able to detect, with a high degree of sophistication, when a child is not progressing the way he or she should be in one or more developmental realms.

Behavioral Strategies for Addressing Common Early Childhood Issues

Although parents may have questions about any number of topics related to early childhood behavior and development, in our experience the "big three" are sleep (e.g., bedtime, sleep training), feeding (e.g., introducing solids, picky eating), and discipline (e.g., handling tantrums and defiance). Furthermore, the bulk of referrals from pediatricians will likely pertain to these topics, as they are the ones that are intentionally raised in each well-child visit, yet, due to constraints on time, frequently given less attention than many parents want or need. Early childhood integrated behavioral health specialists need to know the multiple issues that can arise in each of these general areas at each developmental stage, as well as the behavioral strategies shown to address them most effectively. Ideally, practitioners use accessible language and analogies to convey important behavioral principles (e.g., positive reinforcement) that are important to parenting young children. The use of concrete behavioral tools, such as food or sleep diaries, is also an approach with which specialists should be familiar.

Knowledge of Local Area Resources

Early childhood integrated behavioral health specialists need to be experts at detecting developmental delays or other factors that can derail healthy development, such as family psychosocial stress or parental mental illness. They may not, however, be able to treat these issues if they are quite severe, given the drain on their time and available resources. Therefore, it is essential that these practitioners know where and how to refer young children and their families in need of additional, supplemental services, whether they be the city or county's early intervention program, the preschool special education system, or the local community mental health center. Specialists need to move beyond a mere perfunctory grasp of these systems and to develop relationships with those who work within them, so as to ensure that referrals occur as smoothly and seamlessly as possible.

Basic Clinical Skills

Although not everyone serving as an early childhood integrated behavioral health specialist will have been trained within a formal mental health training program, there are fundamental clinical skills that are nonetheless critical to the work. The crux of the role involves becoming a trusted professional, available to guide families through some very challenging years. To that end, the following are techniques that are indispensable.

(a) *Building Rapport*
    As stated above, the number one goal is to become a trusted resource to the families served by the pediatric practice. The first step toward meeting this goal is to establish a connection with them. Whether you share a favorite color or sports team, finding common ground on which to forge a relationship is a necessary, and highly meaningful, task. Unless you are able to connect with the families you serve in this role, it will be difficult to demonstrate any of the knowledge or other skills on this list.

(b) *Normalizing*

Parents of infants and toddlers are, almost by definition, extremely vulnerable. Though they may know, on an intellectual level, that they are not the first to face the distinct challenges of parenthood, they nonetheless frequently feel that no one could possibly understand or relate to their particular experiences, whether they be internal (e.g., their thoughts about their baby) or external (e.g., their toddler's behavior). Helping a parent to understand on a deep level that feeling frustrated or despairing when a 1-month-old infant cries is *normal*, or that it's *common* for 1-year-olds to hit when they are angry, can be an invaluable service.

(c) *Motivating/Engaging Families*

It is important to remember that parents of infants and toddlers do not always go to their pediatric practice seeking behavioral health services. They may plan to ask the pediatrician a question or two about why their child is acting in a particular way, but, for the most part, they want to be told their child is healthy, get the necessary vaccines, and be on their way. Early childhood integrated behavioral health specialists are in the unique position of needing, in a sense, to "sell their product" to families, and this may not be something that happens quickly or easily. For this reason, we suggest that a familiarity with Motivational Interviewing (Miller & Rollnick, 1991), both theoretically and practically, is essential to the position.

(d) *Balancing Directive vs. Therapeutic Manner*

Early childhood behavioral health specialists are not merely "instructors" providing didactic lectures about infant and toddler development and behavior. On the other hand, they are usually not long-term therapists who do ongoing and in-depth work with a limited caseload of families. Rather, early childhood behavioral health specialists are somewhere in the middle of this spectrum; they need to ensure that families have access to accurate and important information about early childhood, while simultaneously creating a space in which parents feel safe to explore their unique, and often challenging, experiences. Although this "dance" is critical to many of the helping professions, it is especially key to practicing as an integrated behavioral health specialist.

Brief Assessment Skills

At community or outpatient mental health clinics, the intake process typically comprises several steps. There may be an initial phone call, followed by at least one full session—and often more—devoted solely to diagnosing the patient, as well as developing a thorough case conceptualization and appropriate treatment plan. In integrated behavioral health, this is a luxury that we cannot often afford. Patients (or, in the case of infants and toddlers, parents) are not usually coming to their pediatric practice to obtain behavioral health services, and, therefore, such services need to be offered in a straightforward and efficient manner. In addition, the goal is often to see a very large number of patients/families without ever "filling up" on cases and thereby becoming unavailable to pediatricians and families; adopting the typical intake process would quickly make this an impossibility. Rather, within one 45–60-min session, early childhood behavioral health specialists often need to perform a quick assessment of the child/family/situation, develop a case conceptualization, and implement at least one intervention, so that families have something to take home with them. In this way (and this way alone, as the presenting issues are usually very different), an integrated behavioral health specialist needs to operate similarly to a mental health professional working within an emergency setting; even upon first meeting, there is always an eye toward disposition. Although the job often involves treating the patient, there are occasions on which the most effective intervention is to engage in an extensive triage process. Early childhood integrated behavioral health specialists should take great care to assess the urgency of the problem(s) at hand, determine the appropriate points of intervention, and assist the patient/caregivers in getting the right services, whether within the pediatric practice or elsewhere.

The "Integrated Care Backbone"

In our experience, this is one of the most important skill sets that early childhood integrated behavioral health specialists need to master; it is also most difficult to define and explain, in part because it is new to this field (so new, in fact, that we had to make up a name for it). Essentially, until the emergence of integrated behavioral health, pediatricians hesitated to "open Pandora's box" by asking about issues related to behavior and mental health; a primary fear was that patients would disclose important and clinically concerning information that they would then be powerless to address, lacking adequate time, expertise, and resources (Cooper, Valleley, Polaha, Begeny, & Evans, 2006; Horwitz et al., 2007; Perrin & Stancin, 2002; Sugg & Inui, 1992). When behavioral health specialists are, then, integrated into a pediatric practice, the temptation of pediatricians—who are typically busy and overwhelmed as it is—may be to "dump" onto them every single behavioral health issue that crosses their path. And, newly hired integrated behavioral health specialists, eager to prove their utility, frequently agree to accept every single referral—even those that pediatricians have been doing themselves for years (e.g., referrals to Early Intervention). The problem, however, is that if the behavioral health specialist proceeds in this fashion, he or she quickly becomes overwhelmed with referrals, and, over not too much time, is no longer available as a resource to the practice. Additionally, the integrated behavioral health provider must sometimes employ this backbone with patients and parents, who despite clearly needing a higher level of care, prefer to remain in the primary care practice and not be referred out to a more appropriate mental health setting. The "integrated care backbone," therefore, is a necessary tool for ensuring that the integrated behavioral health specialist does not "fill up" the way that a practitioner in a traditional mental health clinic might (and often does). Put slightly differently, the backbone is the characteristic that enables integrated behavioral health specialists to serve the whole practice at any given point in time and in an ongoing manner.

Comprehensive Understanding of the Population Served

If you know one primary care pediatrics practice, you know one primary care pediatrics practice. That is to say, training as an integrated behavioral health specialist generally is limited in its utility unless paired with training focused on the specific needs and issues of the population served by a particular practice. These issues may pertain to a particular cultural or ethnic group (see Chap. 8 by Duch, Germán, & Cuno), or relate to high levels of intergenerational and/or community trauma (see Chap. 2 by Murphy, Dube, Steele & Steele). Practices affiliated with, or close in proximity to, major medical centers may serve a high proportion of children with special medical needs, and it is important for integrated behavioral health specialists to familiarize themselves with the family dynamics that may emerge within these contexts (e.g., fragile child syndrome). Urban practices that serve low-income and minority populations may see high numbers of young children with obesity or asthma, as rates of these disorders are higher in these groups (Bryant-Stephens, 2009; Keet et al., 2015; Nelson, Chiasson, & Ford, 2004; Ogden, Carroll, Kit, & Flegal, 2012; Smith, Hatcher-Ross, Wertheimer, & Kahn, 2005). The more in-depth and nuanced an understanding that an integrated behavioral health specialist has of the population he or she serves, the more effectively he or she can do the work at hand.

Knowledge of Parent–Child Dyadic Interventions

So often when working with infants/toddlers and their families, the patient is neither the child nor the parent. Rather, the patient is the parent–child relationship. Data overwhelmingly suggest, in fact, that a healthy parent–child relationship can serve as a buffer against a host of negative outcomes (Shonkoff, Garner, Committee on Psychosocial Aspects of Child and Family Health, Committee on Early Childhood, Adoption, and Dependent Care, and Section on Developmental and Behavioral Pediatrics et al., 2012; Shonkoff, Boyce, & McEwen, 2009). Integrated early childhood behavioral health specialists are in the unique position of being able to "catch" families when babies are extremely young, as parents of newborns will still make the trip to the pediatrician even when they are not ready to venture anywhere else. Due to the prognostic importance of the parent–child relationship in the first few months and years of life, early childhood integrated behavioral health specialists need to have expertise in therapeutic interventions or techniques shown to build and strengthen this relationship (e.g., Child–Parent Psychotherapy, Lieberman & Van Horn, 2004). Furthermore, specialists need to be able to teach pediatricians—who are even further up on the front lines—to become sophisticated observers of the parent–child relationship, such that they can make the appropriate referrals.

Knowledge of Evidence-Based Treatments for Early Childhood Behavioral Problems

As noted above, the "big three" issues for which young children are referred to early childhood integrated behavioral health specialists are sleep, feeding, and discipline. The latter represents a particularly common issue, as many families who are functioning quite well begin to have difficulties when their toddler starts demonstrating age-appropriate defiance, aggression, and temper tantrums. Even when these behaviors are within normal limits, reflective of the child's developmentally appropriate increasing need for autonomy and control, parents often feel blindsided, and come to their pediatrician seeking help. For this reason, it is essential that early childhood integrated behavioral health specialists have a high degree of familiarity with evidence-based approaches toward young children's disruptive behaviors, such as the approaches used in Parent–Child Interaction Therapy (PCIT, Eyberg, 1999) Incredible Years (Webster-Stratton, 2001) or *1, 2, 3 Magic* (Phelan, 2010). Although whether the specialist would choose, or be able, to administer a full course of treatment would depend on the volume of the practice and the ever-present need to remain available (vs. "filling up"), a facility with the principles and techniques is critical regardless.

How to Talk so Pediatricians will Listen

This heading is indeed a play off the well-known book, *How to Talk so Kids Will Listen & Listen so Kids Will Talk* (Faber & Mazlish, 1980), the idea being that pediatricians usually speak a different language than early childhood behavioral health specialists. In order to communicate effectively, early childhood specialists need to learn aspects of this language, and use it when discussing patient care or other important issues at hand. For example, if an early childhood behavioral health specialist is trained as a psychologist, it is likely that he or she will see families through the lens of attachment theory, and emphasize the importance of parent–child attunement as a necessary condition of subsequent mental health. A pediatrician, however, will likely not be well versed in attachment theory, nor be particularly interested in parent–child attunement when framed in that context. It is incumbent upon the early childhood specialist, therefore, to "translate" these terms and concepts so that they are more accessible to their medical colleagues. In this case, the specialist would do well to speak of the idea of "serve and return" as critical for infant brain development (Shonkoff & Bales, 2011), and the link between these parent–child interactions and not only mental, but also physical health. The more data that early childhood integrated behavioral health specialists can have at their fingertips (e.g., results of the ACEs study, as outlined in this volume by Murphy et al.), the more convincing their case. These data, along with ongoing references to brain development and medical outcomes, will allow pediatricians to move away from historical misconceptions of behavioral health as "touchy-feely" or a "soft science."

Appreciation of the Importance of Universal Screening and a Stepped Care Approach

As mentioned above, one of the most important roles of an early childhood inte-grated behavioral health specialist is to serve a triage function, determining the correct level and points of intervention based on need. This stepped care approach begins with the smallest amount of intervention, and gains in intensity based on assessment of need (Sobell & Sobell, 2000). An efficient and effective way to do this is to implement a universal screening program, whereby all patients in the practice receive developmental and behavioral screens at regular intervals, and then only those patients who score in the at-risk or clinically significant range (or referred by the pediatric provider for other reasons) obtain direct intervention. To this end, early childhood integrated behavioral health specialists need to be famil-iar with the screens administered (e.g., Ages and Stages Questionnaire-3 (ASQ-3; Squires & Bricker, 2009), Ages and Stages Questionnaire: Social-Emotional (ASQ:SE; Squires, Bricker, & Twombly, 2002), and the Modified Checklist for Autism in Toddlers-Revised (MCHAT-R; Robins, Fein, & Barton, 2009)), and to appreciate the extent to which universal screening is critical to the effectiveness of integrated behavioral health.

Interest in Program Development and Ongoing Quality Improvement

As evidenced by many of the items on this list, there is more to being an effective integrated behavioral health specialist than direct service. Even the most skilled clinician will be limited in his or her success in the position without an under-standing of, or interest in, program development and ongoing quality improve-ment. The field of integrated mental healthcare — particularly within pediatrics — is a relatively new one, and so it is basically a guarantee that any practice open to newly incorporating an early childhood integrated behavioral health specialist will need not only the individual specialist per se, but also the creation of the program in which he/she will function. Though direct service with children and families is certainly part of the work, it is also necessary to engage in a range of other tasks, such as the provision of ongoing education to the pediatric providers and practice staff, the creation of screening and referral work flows, and the for-mulation of policies and procedures for optimal program functioning. The effec-tive early childhood integrated behavioral health specialist will see these duties not as burdensome administrative obligations that detract from the "real job" at hand, but, rather, as important responsibilities that have as much — if not more — to do with the overarching goal of improving outcomes for families as direct clinical care.

The "Force" in Workforce

Having outlined the areas of knowledge and particular skill sets for effective early childhood behavioral health specialists, it now becomes possible to ask the second question. That is: who best to be the "force," the individuals most qualified to take on these responsibilities, and most likely to be successful in doing so? To our knowledge, there are four primary groups of professionals who have served, or could successfully serve, in the capacity of early childhood integrated behavioral health specialists: early childhood educators, nurses, paraprofessionals, and mental health providers (psychologists, social workers, counselors, etc.). There are benefits and disadvantages of each within the integrated behavioral health context. In order to determine which type of professional would be the best fit for a particular practice, it is important that some larger questions guide the conversation. Specifically:

1. What is the volume of the pediatric practice?
   A small, family practice with one to two pediatric providers is going to require an early childhood integrated behavioral health specialist with different skills and characteristics than a large practice staffed by over 30 pediatricians and pediatric residents.
2. What are the characteristics of the patient population served?
   Again, depending on the practice population, the demands on—and thus skills needed by—the early childhood integrated behavioral health specialist are going to be quite different. Someone who might excel in the role within a rural or suburban practice that serves primarily those of middle to high socioeconomic status may not do as well in an urban practice with high rates of poverty. It is important to consider these types of patient variables when contemplating the person, or type of person, who will best function in the role.
3. What are the goals of the early childhood integrated behavioral health program?
   It is very important to think about the goals of the early childhood integrated program as a way of determining who will be the best fit for the position. Will the person be expected to do therapeutic interventions with families, or have more of a case management role, perhaps primarily connecting families with outside resources (e.g., Early Intervention)? Will the person be running workshops on particular topics, either for staff or patients? Will the person be implementing a universal screening program, or will someone else be responsible for that task? The only way to choose the right person, or type of person, for the position in a particular practice is for that practice to spend some time and effort really thinking through the details of the job description.

Once these important questions have been answered, the task of choosing the right person for your practice should become much easier. As stated above, there are four groups of professionals that are generally considered to be a good match for these positions, depending on the volume, characteristics, and demands of a particular practice. Below, we go into a bit more detail about considerations to take into account when making the determination for your practice.

Early Childhood Educators Early childhood educators would seem like a natural fit to these positions, for two main reasons. First, they have a true expertise in early childhood, fluent in the numerous developmental milestones that occur in different domains (e.g., cognitive, gross motor, language). Given this, they are very skilled at detecting developmental problems that may arise, even when not yet obvious to a professional with less training in this specific area. Second, early childhood educators are exactly what their name implies: educators. Much of the position of an early childhood integrated behavioral health specialist involves teaching, whether it be the pediatric providers and practice staff (e.g., about the universal screening measures), or the parents of infants and toddlers (e.g., about the importance of talking to your baby or of sleep training). Early childhood educators are both experienced and skilled in this regard. In addition, early childhood educators are generally less expensive to hire than professionals with more extensive training, and, thus, may be advantageous from an economic and financial perspective, if a locality allows for reimbursement of these types of professionals.

On the flip side, however, early childhood educators generally do not have extensive training in dyadic work, or in evidence-based techniques for relationship-based mental health intervention with infants, toddlers, and families. Though very knowledgeable about childhood development and behavior, they may not know the techniques needed to address some of the more complicated and nuanced clinical issues that arise, especially those pertaining more to parental and family dynamics than to children themselves. Early childhood educators also do not have background in brief clinical assessment, or in program development. This is not to say that additional trainings could not be provided, but only that these are the obstacles that may present themselves at baseline.

Nurses Nurses provide a tremendous advantage serving in the position of early childhood integrated behavioral health specialists with regard to their familiarity with the medical setting. Nurses frequently "speak the same language" as pediatric providers and are used to interfacing with medical colleagues. They understand the ways that pediatric practices serve patients (e.g., the schedule of well-child visits), and will likely have a better grasp of how to create successful screening and referral workflows than others of different professional backgrounds. Finally, nurses often rank highest in American surveys of professionals with the highest honesty and ethical standards (Gallup, 2014).

Similar to early childhood educators, however, nurses do not have training in different approaches for how to work with infants, toddlers, and families across a range of issues, particularly those that are more psychologically complex, nor do they generally have backgrounds in brief assessment, or program development. Finally, they may not have extensive background in early childhood behavior and development, as pediatric nurses tend not to specialize in a particular age group.

Paraprofessionals Community Health Workers, Patient Educators, and other paraprofessional members of medical and behavioral health teams have played important roles in the care of patients for decades (Wallace, 1970). Often members of the same community as patients, paraprofessionals may bring enhanced understanding of the cultural and neighborhood level stresses and strengths to the clinical assessment.

As suggested by their title, however, paraprofessionals do not have formal training in their fields, and may be challenged to successfully integrate into the medical setting, to effectively triage levels of need and follow the stepped care approach, and to provide behavioral health services in an evidence-based manner (Mutamba, van Ginneken, Paintain, Wandiembe, & Schellenberg, 2013).

Mental Health Providers: In full disclosure, our program hires our early childhood integrated behavioral health specialists from this pool, and, therefore, we need to acknowledge that this is our bias. We believe that psychologists and licensed clinical social workers (LCSWs) have the training, knowledge, and skills that most closely align with the "checklist" of what successful early childhood integrated behavioral health specialists need to know at a minimum, compiled above. Although individuals may not possess every skill on the list, their backgrounds provide a general context in which additional training can easily fit. For example, it may be that a psychologist has not had formal training in motivational interviewing or a specific evidence-based treatment for early childhood behavioral problems. However, it is likely that these approaches will be in keeping with their clinical training and expertise more generally, such that learning them will not pose a significant challenge. Psychologists are frequently given some training in program development (particularly if they are interested in this field), and both psychologists and LCSWs are often trained in dyadic interventions.

Of course, psychologists and LCSWs are not without their limitations as early childhood integrated behavioral health specialists. As the field is a relatively new one, there are certainly gaps in their training as well. Most notably, many psychology doctoral programs and social work schools do not focus on early childhood, with the exception of perfunctory coverage in general child development courses. The culture of these programs is frequently that psychopathology only starts at age five, and, thus, so too does training in treatment and intervention. In addition, these programs seldom focus on training their students to communicate with professionals from other disciplines. When the term "interdisciplinary" is used, it frequently refers to a treatment team comprising a psychologist, psychiatrist, and social worker (perhaps along with other therapists). Very rarely is a pediatrician, or medical doctor of any sort, included. Therefore, psychologists and LCSWs graduate knowing a language that is very different from that spoken by pediatricians, which presents an important challenge to effective integration within the pediatric setting.

It is clear that different professional backgrounds lend themselves to different parts of the job of early childhood behavioral health specialist. Beyond training or degree, however, there are some personal qualities/characteristics that are beneficial for integrated behavioral health specialists to possess (beyond those that contribute to professional success more generally, of course). These characteristics are listed below and are very important to query about when interviewing potential candidates for these positions.

Flexibility

Within this role, your time is often not your own. Unlike in a more traditional role, you may not be the one to schedule your appointments in a way that suits your preferred daily rhythm. For example, although you may not be a morning person, many parents schedule their babies' well-child visits for first thing in the morning, and so you will need to be available and accessible at that time. Or, you may have planned to catch up on your notes at 3:00 pm on Monday, but it turns out that, just as you're delving into this task, a pediatrician needs for you to meet one of her high-risk families. One of the purposes of being integrated within primary care pediatrics is to be available for "meet and greets," or "warm hand-offs." As these are rarely planned ahead of time, an early childhood integrated behavioral health specialist needs to be flexible with regard to scheduling and to be able to transition between different tasks smoothly and easily. Finally, at practices with higher patient volume, it may be that you need to see multiple families, all of whom are scheduled to see their pediatrician during the same appointment slot.

Preference for (or, at least, tolerance of!) an Open Door

This characteristic is one that is true both literally and figuratively. With regard to the former, early childhood integrated behavioral health specialists need to make active efforts to integrate into the pediatric practice in a palpable and ongoing way. One clear way to do this is to keep one's office door open (when not with patients), thereby communicating availability, and a willingness (or, even, eagerness) to be approached by other members of the practice for consultation. After all, if the ultimate goal is to break down barriers between behavioral and medical health, then removing the physical barrier between them is an important symbolic gesture. On a figurative level, early childhood integrated behavioral health specialists need to demonstrate openness—to collaboration with providers, to continual improvement of systems, and to being pioneers in a relatively new field.

Ability to Work in a Distracting Environment

A primary care pediatric practice – even a relatively small and quiet one– differs a great deal from traditional office environments. Early childhood integrated behavioral health specialists need to be able to focus on their work (whether interactions with patients or more administrative tasks) despite, at times, loud noise (think of children getting vaccines!), interruptions by medical staff, and a generally busy and often frenetic setting. If someone needs a quiet space to be productive, then an integrated care setting may not be a good fit.

On the Ground Example

When we hired Dr. Martin (all names have been changed) to work in one of our busiest practices, we were thrilled with her credentials; she received her degree from a prestigious institution, and had an impressive range of practical experience. We were surprised, therefore, when it became clear that she was struggling in her new position. After some probing, it became clear that she was someone who was able to be most productive when working in a quiet environment, with a closed door; she was finding it difficult to complete her work given the noise and constant bustling of the pediatric primary care environment. We attempted to work with Dr. Martin to put measures into place that would enable her to be more effective, but ultimately, it was clear—to all of us—that the position was not a good fit. And, for our parts, what did we change? Now we *always* ask about this characteristic—whether people can get work done in noisy, busy places—when we interview potential hires!

Ability to Tolerate (and, ideally, surmount) Possible Social Isolation

With only very rare possible exceptions, an early childhood integrated behavioral health specialist will be the only early childhood integrated behavioral health specialist in a given primary care pediatric practice. Although this person may work with numerous colleagues in other fields—pediatricians, nurses, administrative assistants—he or she will have a unique perspective, and a different experience of the patients and practice as a whole. It is important that people hired into these positions feel comfortable in this role, and have the capacity to seek out and find social support among professionals of diverse backgrounds, as well as within networks that may be less geographically convenient, but are accessible via telephone, email, and other methods of communication.

Acceptance of Medical Hierarchy

It is important for integrated behavioral health specialists to keep in the forefront of their minds that the pediatric provider remains paramount within the primary care setting. A colleague of ours once described the goal of the early childhood integrated behavioral health specialist as being "the least irritating irritant." That is to say, no matter how important the behavioral health work is to the well-being of the family at hand, and no matter how well trained the behavioral health specialist is in his or her field, the foremost goal of the pediatric practice is to offer quality pediatric medical care. The integrated behavioral health specialist—even under the most integrated of circumstances!—is a guest in someone else's home, and the psycho-social interventions will never take precedence over the medical care sought by patients.

On the Ground Example

One of our early childhood behavioral health specialists sought peer supervision after what she experienced as a very negative interaction with a pediatrician. The specialist, Ms. Clark, found Dr. Davis, a pediatrician, in the hallway of the practice, and attempted to speak with her about a recent session with a shared patient. Ms. Clark perceived Dr. Davis to be distracted and dismissive and was personally offended by her demeanor. When we advised Ms. Clark to process the exchange with Dr. Davis directly, however, Dr. Davis apologized, and explained that when Ms. Clark had approached her in the hallway, she had just finished transferring a patient under severe respiratory distress to the emergency room. She was indeed distracted, but not for any reason having to do with behavioral health! From that point forward, Ms. Clark always remembered that pediatricians are often involved in life or death situations and judgment calls; though behavioral health is critical for long-term health outcomes, it is seldom an acute crisis in the same way. Consequently, for good reason, in a medical setting, it will almost always be a secondary priority.

Passion for the Cause

Admittedly, this last quality may sound a bit hokey, but we suggest that it is quite important. Although the same could be said of many jobs, being an early childhood integrated behavioral health specialist is not easy. In many ways, it is far less challenging to serve in a more traditional capacity, where the structure and protocols are well established, and there is little room for change. In contrast, integrated pediatric behavioral health is a relatively new field, rife with opportunities for innovation. For reasons discussed elsewhere in this volume (e.g., universal access, "pro-stigma,") we believe wholeheartedly that this model of care is a critical addition to the behavioral health landscape, and for many patients, may be preferable to service delivery models that have historically been more prevalent (e.g., outpatient mental health clinics). It is precisely this belief that has fueled us when hurdles have arisen, and resistance—whether on the part of individual providers or greater systems—has reared its head. Arguably, those taking on these positions need to possess this devotion to the principles behind the integrated care model in order to remain committed and diligent even in the face of abundant obstacles.

The "Development" in Workforce Development

We have now completed our discussion of the "work" and the "force" aspects of workforce development. We have expounded upon the various tasks and skills that comprise the role of an early childhood integrated behavioral health specialist, as well as the types of professional backgrounds and personal traits/qualities that we believe will most lend themselves to success in this field. We now turn to the very realistic possibility that no one hired into this position will possess all of these abilities and qualities at the outset and that ongoing training and honing of skills will be both necessary and important. In our experience, there are three areas that merit the most attention in this regard.

The first of these areas is Motivational Interviewing (MI). As stated above, a familiarity with this approach (Miller & Rollnick, 1991), both theoretically and practically, is extremely beneficial to working within an integrated care setting. This is true because families do not always come to primary care pediatrics expecting behavioral health services, and thus may not fully "buy in" to the importance of behavioral health. In addition, resistance on the part of pediatricians is not an uncommon phenomenon, and early childhood integrated behavioral health specialists need to be able to address this effectively (and calmly!). Although it is possible to obtain an understanding of MI by reading the myriad materials available or by attending a formal training, in our experience the skills are only fully learned (as is often the case) when practiced in an ongoing manner. Therefore, our group has established a monthly MI practice group, during which case examples are discussed, and group members participate in role plays.

The second area in need of ongoing attention is the development of an "Integrated Care Backbone," which is continually challenging for early childhood behavioral health specialists. At times, it appears to be in conflict with the third area, to which we refer as "Integration into the Culture of the Practice." These two tasks—to set firm limits with families and pediatricians while still assimilating well into the practice—need to occur simultaneously, and there is a tendency for early childhood integrated behavioral health specialists to allow the pendulum to swing too far in one direction or the other. It is important that both of these skills be assessed in a continuing manner, and addressed by supervisors as needed. Again, practicing (e.g., via role plays) may be very helpful here, in addition to reflective individual supervision. For example, if someone is typically a "people-pleaser," then he or she may have a difficult time saying "no" to a pediatrician, and will need concrete assistance in coming up with appropriate backbone language and tolerating the resulting anxiety. This language may include training a pediatrician on the best way to make a referral, for example, providing specific concerns, rather than a mere phrase such as, "this family is a mess." Would a pediatrician ever refer to a pulmonologist stating only that the child's "breathing is kind of a nightmare?" No. These analogies can be very useful to introduce into the dialogue.

On the Ground Example

In August of 2014, we hired several new psychologists to serve as integrated behavioral health specialists at different pediatric practices within our network. Three months later, upon reviewing various metrics, we noticed that Dr. Denton had three times as many referrals as his colleagues; he was swamped, and was scheduling patients 6–8 weeks in advance, a time frame that — though perhaps typical for urban community mental health clinics — is not in keeping with the integrated care model. Upon further probing, we saw that Dr. Denton was accepting every single referral he received, no matter how sparse (e.g., "child seems sad") or inappropriate for our model (e.g., "child needs a neuropsychological evaluation"). Dr. Denton then acknowledged that he had a very difficult time saying no to people and that the act went against his "people-pleasing nature" in a way that felt very uncomfortable for him. We were able to work closely with Dr. Denton on developing his "Integrated Care Backbone," which included a range of experiential exercises, such as role plays and concrete direction to his pediatric colleagues regarding the nature of appropriate referrals. Dr. Denton is still with us, has been very successful, and is currently no more swamped than any of his colleagues!

Finally, we turn to integration into the culture of the practice. Although it is critical to address the ongoing training needs of the integrated early childhood behavioral health specialist, it is also necessary to focus on training and education of the entire pediatric practice team. In other words, if the goal is to create actual integrated care, then all members of the practice — pediatricians, nurses, administrative assistants — will need some training as well. Within this context, an expert workgroup was convened at the 2013 Patient-Centered Medical Home Research Conference, the task of which was to recommend policies that would promote integrated behavioral healthcare (Ader et al., 2015). One of their primary recommendations was the development of "interdisciplinary training systems to support each member" of the integrated care team (p. 915). The content of these trainings would likely vary among different types of settings. In our setting, for example, which is characterized by high levels of family and community trauma, we focus a great deal on the impact of toxic stress on the developing brain, and the extent to which a healthy parent–child attachment is able to buffer these effects (Shonkoff, Garner, Committee on Psychosocial Aspects of Child and Family Health, Committee on Early Childhood, Adoption, and Dependent Care, & Section on Developmental and Behavioral Pediatrics et al., 2012; Briggs et al., 2014). The goal is to provide pediatricians with a framework through which to observe the parent–child relationship within the exam room, so that referrals to the early childhood integrated behavioral health specialist are most appropriate. Other topics of our training curriculum include ways to assess psychosocial stressors so as to be able to predict the likelihood of a developmental delay (vs. waiting for the delay itself), ensuring that pediatricians convey the same confidence when "prescribing" a behavioral intervention as they do when prescribing antibiotics (with the same inclusion of details about time frame, appropriate expectations, etc.), and "spiels" pediatricians can use to address common early childhood issues prior to making a referral to the specialist. We have included a sampling of these "spiels" below.

Sample "Spiels"

1. Illustrating "the power of attention" to parents of defiant or disruptive toddlers:
   "Tell the patient's mother that her **attention is like money**—she needs to think of it as payment. To illustrate, present the following scenario, or one like it: I get to work every day around 9 am. Let's say that tomorrow I get in at 8 am, and my boss sees me in the hallway and says, 'Wow, you're so awesome to get here so early,' and then takes out her wallet and gives me a $100 bill. Do you think I'd get here at 8 am the next day? Why? Exactly. Because we ALL—not only kids— do things we get rewarded for. Money is a huge reward for grown-ups. What's the biggest reward for kids? Attention. So every time you give your child attention, you are paying her, and whatever she did that got attention, she is going to do again. You have to think to yourself: do I want to pay my child for this? Do I want her to do it again?"

2. Describing how to optimize brain development to parents of infants:
   "You can think about your baby's brain development the way you think of a game of tennis, or of catch. The way he learns is to serve the ball, or to throw it at you. What does this look like? Well, he makes a sound, or he gestures toward something, or he makes a funny face. The best way to help his brain develop (which is basically another way to say help him get smarter) is to return the ball, or—if you're not into tennis—to catch it and throw it back. So, YOU make a sound back at him, or a gesture, or a funny face. Believe it or not, these are the very first "conversations" that you are having with your baby, and they are so, so, so important. So much of the pleasure for him is about connecting with you—by showing him that you hear him by throwing that ball back, you're telling him that you understand him, and starting to build those really important brain connections."

3. Explaining to parents how best to respond to normal tantrums:
   "First, tell the patient's father to reflect his child's emotion: for example, 'I can see you are very frustrated right now.' He should not belittle the tantrum or the reason behind it (for example, 'Oh come on, it's just a cookie! Get over it!'), as that will only make it worse. If the father doesn't seem to get this, ask about the last time he had a bad day. Would it have helped to calm him down if someone said it was no big deal? Second, have the father ignore the behavior—not in a mean way, but in an I'm-not-going-to-pay-attention-to-this-because-I-don't-want-to-encourage-it way. He might even say something like, 'I am going to go read a book; I'd love for you to come read with me when you calm down.' And then he needs to go read that book—chances are, his little one will be right on his heels!"

When we talk about training the pediatric providers, however (and, in our case, the pediatric residents), it is important to remember that this training does not only occur in one direction. For example, many of our early childhood integrated behavioral health specialists were shocked to discover that pediatricians are not taught attachment theory (Ainsworth & Bowlby, 1991; Bowlby, 1969) in medical school or during residency. How could pediatricians—particularly those practicing in an underserved, urban area such as the Bronx—be unaware of how to ascertain the quality of the relationship between children and their caregivers, especially when disturbances in this relationship are so important from a prognostic standpoint?

During one interdisciplinary team training (aimed to increase the ability of psychologists to understand the pediatricians' perspective, and vice versa), this bafflement was posed to a very experienced pediatrician, who concurred that the topic would ideally be incorporated into the medical school curriculum in the future. Several minutes later, this same pediatrician referenced "RSV." The integrated behavioral health specialists looked puzzled, even when the pediatrician spelled out the diagnosis: Respiratory Syncytial Virus. Now, RSV is, per WebMD, "a common and highly contagious virus that infects the respiratory tract of most children before their second birthday," and, in a group of several *early childhood* behavioral health specialists working *within a pediatric setting*, no one knew what it was.

We bring up this story to highlight the need for true interdisciplinary training. If we are striving to achieve genuinely integrated care, this means not only that pediatric providers need to learn more about early childhood behavioral health, but also that early childhood behavior health specialists need to learn more about common medical diagnoses. The point is that the two fields have been falsely separated for too long, and only by integrating them will young children and their families be able to obtain the holistic care they need and deserve.

On the Ground Example

How do we teach pediatricians about attachment theory, given its integral role in the social and emotional development of young children? By explaining to them that a well-child visit is like a miniature lab, in which a version of the "Strange Situation" (Ainsworth, Blehar, Waters, & Wall, 1978) plays out repeatedly. We train pediatricians to become "sophisticated observers of attachment" by looking closely at the parent–child dyad during moments of distress—for example, during infant ear exams (all kids hate ear exams!), or when toddlers are told they are going to need vaccines. Pediatricians are told to notice whether the child looks toward the parent, whether the parent responds, and, ultimately, whether the parent's actions are effective in soothing the child. If, based on these pieces of "data," the pediatrician detects the presence of an insecure attachment, then he or she is instructed to make a referral to the early childhood integrated behavioral health specialist—preferably in the form of a warm handoff!

A final point with regard to workforce development, and one that brings together all three parts of the matter at hand—the work, the force, and the development. Namely, it is important that early childhood integrated behavioral health specialists continually view their work through a quality improvement (QI) lens. The field of integrated behavioral healthcare within primary care pediatrics is still in its infancy, and so there is no established manual for how this is done (hence, this book!). Furthermore, as elaborated above, there is no "one size fits all," and so, by definition, an early childhood integrated behavioral health specialist beginning work in a new practice will always, in some senses, be starting from scratch. There needs to be a constant eye toward evaluating, and subsequently finding ways to improve, the systems and processes that allow us to offer the best care to children and families. Examples include—but are far from limited to—making sure that as many children are being screened as possible, all pediatricians in a practice are referring to and utilizing the behavioral health resources in an effective manner, and behavioral health specialists are thinking creatively and flexibly about the services they offer. If a medical center includes multiple sites, then this QI lens is important both for individual practice success and for ensuring that systems are sustainable and replicable across settings.

The field of early childhood integrated behavioral health is a nascent one, requiring significant thought related to models of intervention, methods of evaluation, and workforce development. We hope that this chapter outlines the various workforce development aspects we believe key for success in these exciting roles.

References

Ader, J., Stille, C. J., Keller, D., Miller, B. F., Barr, M. S., & Perrin, J. M. (2015). The medical home and integrated behavioral health: Advancing the policy agenda. *Pediatrics, 135*(5), 909–917.

Ainsworth, M. D. S., Blehar, M. C., Waters, E., & Wall, S. (1978). *Patterns of attachment: A psychological study of the strange situation.* Hillsdale, NJ: Erlbaum.

Ainsworth, M. D. S., & Bowlby, J. (1991). An ethological approach to personality development. *American Psychologist, 46*, 331–341.

Bowlby, J. (1969). *Attachment and loss* (Attachment, Vol. 1). New York, NY: Basic Books.

Briggs, R. D., Silver, E. J., Krug, L. M., Mason, Z. S., Schrag, R. D. A., Chinitz, S., & Racine, A. D. (2014). Healthy Steps as a moderator: The impact of maternal trauma on child social-emotional development. *Clinical Practice in Pediatric Psychology, 2*(2), 166–175.

Bryant-Stephens, T. (2009). Asthma disparities in urban environments. *Journal of Allergy and Clinical Immunology, 123*(6), 1199–1206.

Cooper, S., Valleley, R. J., Polaha, J., Begeny, J., & Evans, J. H. (2006). Running out of time: Physician management of behavioral health concerns in rural pediatric primary care. *Pediatrics, 118*(1), e132–e138.

Eyberg, S. M (1999). Parent-child interaction therapy: Integrity checklists and session materials. Retrieved July 20, 2015, from www.pcit.org

Faber, A., & Mazlish, E. (1980). *How to talk so kids will listen and listen so kids will talk.* New York, NY: Avon Books.

Gallup. (2014). Honesty and ethics in professions. Retrieved July 19, 2015, from http://www.gallup.com/poll/1654/honesty-ethics-professions.aspx2014

Horwitz, S. M., Kelleher, K. J., Stein, R. E., Storfer-Isser, A., Youngstrom, E. A., Park, E. R., … & Hoagwood, K. E. (2007). Barriers to the identification and management of psychosocial issues in children and maternal depression. *Pediatrics, 119*(1), e208–e218.

Keet, C. A., McCormack, M. C., Pollack, C. E., Peng, R. D., McGowan, E., & Matsui, E. C. (2015). Neighborhood poverty, urban residence, race/ethnicity, and asthma: Rethinking the inner-city asthma epidemic. *Journal of Allergy and Clinical Immunology, 135*(3), 655–662.

Lieberman, A. F., & Van Horn, P. (2004). *Don't hit my mommy!: A manual for child-parent psychotherapy with young witnesses of family violence.* Washington, DC: Zero to Three.

Miller, W. R., & Rollnick, S. (1991). *Motivational interviewing: Preparing people to change addictive behavior.* New York, NY: Guilford Press.

Mutamba, B. B., van Ginneken, N., Paintain, L. S., Wandiembe, S., & Schellenberg, D. (2013). Roles and effectiveness of lay community health workers in the prevention of mental, neurological and substance use disorders in low and middle income countries: A systematic review. *BMC Health Services Research, 13*(1), 412.

Nelson, J. A., Chiasson, M. A., & Ford, V. (2004). Childhood overweight in a New York City WIC population. *American Journal of Public Health, 94*(3), 458–462.

Ogden, C. L., Carroll, M. D., Kit, B. K., & Flegal, K. M. (2012). Prevalence of obesity and trends in body mass index among US children and adolescents, 1999–2010. *JAMA, 307*(5), 483–490.

Perrin, E., & Stancin, T. (2002). A continuing dilemma: Whether and how to screen for concerns about children's behavior. *Pediatrics in review/American Academy of Pediatrics, 23*(8), 264–276.

Phelan, T. (2010). *1-2-3 magic: Effective discipline for children 2–12.* Glen Ellyn, IL: ParentMagic.

Robins, D. L., Fein, D., & Barton, M. (2009). The modified checklist for autism in toddlers. Revised (M-CHAT-R). Self-published.

Shonkoff, J. P., & Bales, S. N. (2011). Science does not speak for itself: Translating child development research for the public and its policymakers. *Child Development, 82,* 17–32.

Shonkoff, J. P., Garner, A. S., The Committee on Psychosocial Aspects of Child and Family Health, Committee on Early Childhood, Adoption, and Dependent Care, and Section on Developmental and Behavioral Pediatrics, Siegel, B. S., Dobbins, M. I., et al. (2012). The lifelong effects of early childhood adversity and toxic stress. *Pediatrics, 129*(1), 1–35.

Shonkoff, J. P., Boyce, W. T., & McEwen, B. S. (2009). Neuroscience, molecular biology, and the childhood roots of health disparities: Building a new framework for health promotion and disease prevention. *JAMA: Journal of the American Medical Association, 301,* 2252–2259.

Smith, L. A., Hatcher-Ross, J. L., Wertheimer, R., & Kahn, R. S. (2005). Rethinking race/ethnicity, income, and childhood asthma: Racial/ethnic disparities concentrated among the very poor. *Public Health Reports, 120*(2), 109–116.

Sobell, M. B., & Sobell, L. C. (2000). Stepped care as a heuristic approach to the treatment of alcohol problems. *Journal of Consulting and Clinical Psychology, 68*(4), 573.

Squires, J., & Bricker, D. (2009). *Ages and stages questionnaires, third edition (ASQ-3).* Baltimore, MD: Paul H. Brookes.

Squires, J., Bricker, D., & Twombly, E. (2002). *Ages and stages questionnaire: Social-emotional (ASQ:SE).* Baltimore, MD: Paul H. Brookes.

Sugg, N. K., & Inui, T. (1992). Primary care physicians' response to domestic violence: Opening Pandora's box. *JAMA, 267*(23), 3157–3160.

Wallace, H. (1970). The Paraprofessional Mental Health Workers: What Are We All About? Presented at American Orthopsychiatric Association meeting, San Francisco, CA, March, 1970.

Webster-Stratton, C. (2001). The Incredible Years: Parents, teachers, and children training series. *Residential Treatment for Children & Youth, 18*(3), 31–45.

Chapter 7
Healthy Steps at Montefiore: Our Journey from Start Up to Scale

Rahil D. Briggs, Rebecca Schrag Hershberg, and Miguelina Germán

Abstract With a decade of experience in integrated early childhood behavioral health programming, we present our lessons learned from Montefiore. We begin with our program model and chart the progression of the model as we expanded. We note why we made certain changes to the model, and how taking the model to scale throughout our system required modifications. We share our top three lessons learned: breaking down silos while respecting the medical hierarchy, navigating thorny issues of privacy related to documentation and communication, and the need to battle isolation as integrated behavioral health providers.

Keywords Healthy Steps • Montefiore • Integrated early childhood behavioral health • Pediatrics

Introduction

Montefiore Medicine has been a pioneer in early childhood integrated behavioral health. After a year of pilot programming, we formally became a Healthy Steps program in 2006, and have accumulated over a decade of experience in this arena. In this chapter, we will describe our program model, detail the mistakes we made (so that you can hopefully avoid them), and review lessons learned along the way, as we expanded our program from one initial primary care practice in 2005 to 19 in 2016.

R.D. Briggs, Psy.D. (✉) • R.S. Hershberg, Ph.D. • M. Germán, Ph.D.
Montefiore Health System, Bronx, NY, USA
e-mail: rabriggs@montefiore.org; drschrag@littlehousecalls.com; mgerman@montefiore.org

© Springer International Publishing Switzerland 2016   105
R.D. Briggs (ed.), *Integrated Early Childhood Behavioral Health in Primary Care*, DOI 10.1007/978-3-319-31815-8_7

Program Model

Setting, Population, and Design

Montefiore Medical Group (MMG) is a division of Montefiore Health System, the University Hospital for Albert Einstein College of Medicine, and provides medical care to residents of the Bronx and lower Westchester County through a network of 19 pediatric primary care practices, community health centers, and urgent care sites. These sites currently serve more than 90,000 children, 1/3 of whom fall in the birth−5 age range ($N \approx 35,000$). Approximately 75 % of these children have Medicaid insurance, and almost 80 % identify as Hispanic and/or Black.

Although Healthy Steps (HS) has traditionally focused on developmental and procedural outcomes and HS Specialists (HSSs) are often early childhood educators or nurses, HS at Montefiore deviates from the usual model in two ways. First, we place significant emphasis on the social emotional development of young children *and* the mental health of their caregivers, and second, we do this by employing licensed clinical social workers and licensed psychologists. For more on the traditional Healthy Steps program, please see Chap. 5 in this volume.

Our program has two tracks: Development and Behavior (DB) Consults and Intensive Services (IS). In DB consults, ongoing universal behavioral health screenings and/or pediatricians' concerns result in referrals to Healthy Steps Specialists for assessment and short-term interventions on a range of topics, including (but not limited to) sleep, feeding, and discipline. In Intensive Services, we identify children at risk for a host of negative outcomes related to psychosocial stress as early as possible and enroll them and their caregivers to receive preemptive behavioral health services until the child turns 5 years old. As mentioned above, our staff are licensed clinical social workers or psychologists, each of whom have expertise in early childhood mental health, parent–child dyadic work, and adult mental health issues. Please see Chap. 6 on workforce development for more information.

Screenings

Our goal is to universally screen all the young children and their parents in the medical practice. We accomplish this through a team-based approach focused on obtaining screenings during well-child visits. Screenings are generally parent completed, scored by nursing staff, entered into our electronic medical record (EMR), and reviewed by pediatricians. We have configured our EMR to prompt medical staff when a certain screening is due and to automatically score those screening tools when possible (e.g., copyright protections allow).

To identify children at risk at the earliest possible moment, we administer the Adverse Childhood Experiences, or ACEs screening tool (Felitti et al., 1998). The ACEs study demonstrated the impact of traumatic childhood experiences (including abuse, neglect, and household dysfunction) on a range of health outcomes. In addition, these same traumatic experiences are known to impact parenting via a range of pathways (Murphy et al., 2013). It is our hypothesis, therefore, that parental ACEs scores may be the best way to identify newborn babies at risk for social emotional problems.

Between the prenatal period and age 4 months, ACEs screenings are completed by parents (or expectant parents) and returned to the primary care provider. We use a form that asks parents simply to endorse the number of ACEs they've experienced, rather than endorse the specific items. Once the child is born, we also ask parents to report on the child's ACEs, in the same manner (total score).

Lesson Learned: In our first site, we offered IS enrollment to *all* first time parents. We initially believed this was an effective way to provide the program to young parents who were most likely to have questions and be unsure or overwhelmed about parenting. Although that was indeed true, it was also the case that we were not able to enroll many high-risk families due to their already having a child. Moreover, we found our pediatric residents (who were also parents using the practice for medical care) enrolled in the program as well. While we appreciated endorsement of the program, it was not the best use of limited resources due to the residents' notably lower risk status.

In our second site, we developed a risk checklist, based on the literature on the impact of psychosocial stressors on child social–emotional development. We attempted to teach the pediatricians about the major risk factors for poor social emotional outcomes in children, such as having a parent with mental illness, homelessness, and teen pregnancy. That practice proceeded to generate fewer referrals than expected (and desired), which we attributed to the idea that a baby's risk status, measured in this manner, was too nebulous a concept for many pediatricians to reliably assess.

As a result of the above experiences, we began using the ACEs screening as a tool for enrollment at our third site in 2013. The screening is short, connected to health outcomes, and we find that parents are open to completing it. Our ACEs screening is introduced by a letter, and allows parents to simply report their total number, without endorsing specific ACEs (our data suggest that this encourages more honest responses, and also alleviates some provider concern re: events that would otherwise be reportable for abuse or neglect reasons). Please see the Appendix for a copy of our ACEs screening.

Any pregnant mother with an ACEs score of 4 or more is automatically referred to our program, introduced to the HSS, and offered enrollment in the Intensive Services track. If a mother did not visit a Montefiore OB/GYN practice with ACEs screenings, the same screening is conducted during the first few months of visits in Pediatrics (exact visit is determined by each site). During these visits, mothers, fathers, or other caregivers complete an ACEs screening both regarding their own childhood and the childhood of their newborn. Although it may seem unlikely for a newborn to have ACEs, this is, sadly, not an uncommon scenario in the Bronx. For example, an infant born to a single, depressed mother and whose father is in prison enters the world with an ACEs score of three. It is critical that we track babies' ACEs so that we can make all efforts to keep the number below the threshold of four that is associated with vastly increased risk of negative outcomes over time (see chapter by Dr. Murphy et al. in this volume for further detail). We believe that the ACEs screening is our best approach for early identification of families at risk. First, by screening the parents' ACEs we are not waiting for a child to screen positive on a risk assessment before intervening (in a previous study with a very at risk sample, only 8 % of infants in the practice screened positive on the Ages and Stages Questionnaire: Social Emotional at the 6 month visit (Briggs et al., 2012)). Second, we are not overextending enrollment slots due to offering it to an entire, preselected group (such as first time parents). In a world of limited resources, such overextension can doom a program. Instead, we are using this brief screening, with well-documented long-term implications, and identifying children at risk either prenatally or within the first 4 months of life.

If IS enrollment is declined when the program is first offered, there are additional universal screenings for maternal depression conducted by the pediatrician at children's 2-month and 24-month well-child pediatric visits. In addition, young children are universally screened for the presence of social emotional problems, autism, and general development at multiple pediatric visits during their first 3 years. These additional screens provide multiple opportunities for young children in need to be identified for treatment. Although a poor score on the screening tools suggests to primary care providers that the child should perhaps be referred to HS, pediatricians and nursing staff are encouraged to use their own clinical judgment to refer young children and/or their caregivers to our program for any relevant reason. Although we accept IS referrals only until the child's 18-month visit, behavior and development consultations are available through age 5.

Our screening schedule:

Newborn: Parental and child ACEs
2 months: Patient Health Questionnaire-2 (PHQ-2; parental depression)
12 months: Ages and Stages Questionnaire-3 (ASQ-3)
18 months: Modified Checklist of Autism in Toddlers, Revised (MCHAT-R)
24 months: Ages and Stages Questionnaire: Social Emotional (ASQ:SE), PHQ-2
36 months: ASQ:SE
48 months: Patient Symptom Checklist-17 (PSC-17) (Jellinek et al., 1988)
60 months: PSC-17

> **Lesson Learned:** Screening tools must be short, written at an appropriate reading level, easy to score, and available in the languages your patients speak. Ideally, they are also normed on a population similar to that being screened. While some program designers exert a great deal of time and energy determining which screening tool to use, we believe a better approach is to simply determine the best fit for your practice, knowing that the most important part of the process is simply getting the conversation started. After all, a screening tool is merely that: a screening tool. A concerning score is not an end in and of itself; rather, it merely prompts both the pediatrician and/or the HSS to do a more comprehensive assessment.

Clinical Services and Interventions

Development and Behavior Consults

- Children are referred for DB consults by pediatricians, other practice staff (e.g., nurses), or parents generally due to a particular issue that presents itself during a pediatric visit (e.g., behavior, feeding problems, need for sleep training).
- Children 0–5 can be referred (5th birthday is the cutoff).
- Interventions with these children can be done in an exam room, in the HS office right after the visit, or by scheduling follow-up appointments for them to see the HSS on another day. Sessions range in length from 15 min (e.g., in an exam room following MD visit) to 60 min (e.g., separately scheduled session).
- If possible, a child ACEs is done in order to assess trauma history.
- Generally, this is short-term treatment and we schedule no more than 4–5 visits at a given time for a particular issue (e.g., once a week for a month). Children/families who need more intensive services should be referred out for additional help.

  - However, a new issue a few months later can result in a new referral.

- Children who are seen for a DB consult and are under 18 months may be enrolled in the Intensive Services program if deemed appropriate.
- It is very important to close the loop with the referring medical provider with regard to final action/outcome. Elsewhere in this volume, our pediatrician colleagues (Brown, Bloomfield, and Warman) detail the common lament of pediatricians that they "never hear back after a mental health referral." We advise our HSS to always route the medical provider the following:

  - Documentation of first outreach to the family (which acknowledges the referral),
  - The first clinical note,
  - Important disposition information (e.g., to outside services).

Intensive Services

- Babies whose caregivers have 4 or more ACEs, per universal screening, are automatically referred to the Intensive Services (IS) program and offered enrollment. Babies can also be referred by social work or medical providers based on other risk variables, be siblings of children already in IS, or be children whom a HSS saw for a DB consult. Any child referred before (or at) 18 months is eligible for Intensive Services, and HSS use their judgment as to when to enroll.

Lesson learned: We have worked hard to advise HSS not to "over enroll." As much as the Intensive Services program would likely benefit every family, it is also quite time- and labor intensive, and so patient slots need to be saved for those most in need.

- IS babies are seen at every possible well-child visit, either in a co-managed visit with both the pediatrician and HSS, or in a visit with the HSS before or after the pediatric visit. A child has 15 well-child visits during the first 5 years of life (American Academy of Pediatrics, 2008). Ongoing interventions concentrate on promoting secure attachment, developmental guidance, experiences of caregiver trauma and the impact on the child, and general behavioral intervention with a focus on positive parenting and nonphysical discipline. Interventions are generally offered as part of the well-child visit; if needed, however, families may return for separate follow-up visits with their HSS.
- HSS are informed that the patient's visit is scheduled with the pediatrician via a report that is generated by our EMR.

Lesson Learned: We have experimented in the past with asking parents to make two appointments, one for the PCP and one for the HSS, back to back, when they were scheduling, but parents found this laborious and thus it was not done consistently.

- Babies enrolled in IS receive the following *additional screenings*:

  - Follow-up child ACEs at 12-, 24-, 36-, 48-, and 60 months of age

- Children/families participate in IS until the child's 5th year well-child visit
- We advise HSS to remain in contact with the child's pediatrician and work as a team as needed. If a HSS knows he/she is going to miss a well-child visit for any reason, we ask them to inform the child's pediatrician, and provide outreach to family if deemed necessary.
- Children "graduate" early IF:

- Two screenings in a row are not elevated,
- AND they are doing very well in the clinical judgment of the HSS (this can be sufficient even if the screenings are high—for example, if the child has a developmental delay, but the family is highly intact and the child is receiving appropriate services).
- Early graduates are informed that the HS specialist will not be preemptively seeing them at their well-child visits anymore, but are always available should questions/concerns arise. This is framed as an accomplishment, based on how well the child is doing, and how effectively caregivers are parenting. A standard letter is available to document early graduation if desired.

- *IS Dropouts*
  - Children under 2 years are considered to be dropouts if they have not been at the practice for 12 months.
  - Children over 2 years are considered dropouts if they have not been at the practice for 18 months.

> **Lesson Learned**: keeping track of HS IS dropouts has been a challenge, for a few reasons. At several practices, hundreds of families are enrolled, and it is a difficult task for HSS to monitor who is due and/or overdue for a well-child visit. We have experimented with various systems for achieving this (e.g., spread sheets, alerts in our EMR), and, in the interest of full disclosure, are still honing the process. Part of the challenge in our particular medical system is that our patient population is quite transient. We serve a large immigrant population (i.e., families who are still in the process of finding where they will make their permanent home), as well as families whose phone numbers often change, and who move frequently. Most of our dropouts stem from these causes; that is, families leave the pediatric practice as a whole. It is only exceedingly rare that a family continues to receive medical care at one of our pediatric practices, but opts out of participating in the HS IS track.

It is important to establish criteria regarding early graduation and defining when a family has "dropped out," to ensure that these coveted slots are occupied by the families most in need, and to ensure the program is designed to release slots that are not being used.

Parental Mental Health

One of the earliest lessons we learned when implementing our early childhood integrated behavioral health program was that the brief parenting interventions we offered did not appear to be effective when parents had their own significant mental health challenges. As discussed above, many of the caregivers with whom we work have severe trauma histories, and it is not uncommon that these mothers experienced Posttraumatic Stress Disorder (PTSD) symptoms—either for the first time or as a relapse—within the context of having and raising a baby. Other mothers experience postpartum depression and/or anxiety symptoms, and still others have prior psychiatric diagnoses (e.g., Bipolar Disorder) for which they are in need of treatment. Regardless of the particular symptoms or diagnosis at hand, we have found that offering psychoeducation and parenting strategies without addressing these parental mental health (PMH) issues is, at best, unsuccessful, and at worst, counterproductive or even harmful. Given this, we made a decision early on to invest substantial resources in our two-generation Healthy Steps Parental Mental Health program. For caregivers who present with mental health symptoms, specialized HS staff are available to provide ongoing individual psychotherapy and, if needed, psychotropic medication within the pediatric outpatient setting. We believe that integration of an adult mental health provider increases the likelihood that pediatricians will screen for maternal depression and ACEs, that caregivers will follow through on the referral, and that caregivers will attend counseling sessions.

A few notes on the concrete details of how the PMH aspect of our program works:

- Caregivers of children under the age of 5 may be eligible to participate in our Parental Mental Health Program (PMH), through which they are able to receive long-term, evidence-informed therapy. Ideally, the child of a parent receiving PMH services is enrolled in our HS Intensive Services track, although this is not always possible.
- Parents are encouraged to have a primary care provider in the network to ensure collaborative care, and this is a process with which our staff assists.
- Referrals for PMH are made to the Healthy Steps Specialists who coordinate outreach and refer to alternative agencies if a parent cannot be seen on site, due to insurance or scheduling limitations.
- PMH providers document in both the parent's and child's chart that patient is actively receiving mental health services through HS to alert pediatricians of treatment. However, PMH services are then documented in parent's chart in accordance with legal and privacy rules.

Education of Medical Colleagues

In addition to the clinical services provided to young children and their families, HS at Montefiore also engages in significant educational efforts. Although we believe that education will need to be an important part of the job for most (if not all) early childhood integrated behavioral health specialists, this is clearly more the case in primary care practices affiliated with medical schools and residency programs. Through both formal didactics and informal case consultation, HS staff members teach medical students, pediatric residents, and attending physicians. The medical students and residents participate in a 2-h introductory lecture, and then each spends an afternoon shadowing a HSS during patient visits. The lecture addresses early childhood brain development within a relationship context, attachment theory, toxic stress, and best practices for engaging with caregivers around issues of discipline and child development. In addition, the HS staff regularly present at staff meetings and engage in quality improvement projects designed to improve screening and referral rates of young children and their caregivers.

Lessons We Have Learned

Although we've done our best to highlight certain "lessons learned" in our program description, the ones discussed below are more global in nature, and merit a more detailed treatment given their nuances and complexities. It bears emphasis that integrated early childhood care brings unique challenges. Previously unforeseen questions emerge when thinking about, for example, how much of a parent's information to include in a baby's chart, and how to ensure that the pediatrician is appropriately informed about a parent's history. The three most challenging areas to consider are breaking down silos while respecting the medical home, documentation/communication/privacy, and isolation of behavioral health providers.

Lesson #1: Breaking Down Silos While Respecting the Hierarchy

In order to fully integrate an early childhood behavioral health program into a primary care setting, a system-wide paradigm shift had to occur. From security guards to the front desk staff, nursing, pediatricians, and our patients, we have needed to engage in ongoing education and discourse. For example, the security desk needed to be informed that "Healthy Steps" is a program within pediatrics, and that, even if an adult caregiver comes in alone for his or her PMH session, he/she will be registered in the pediatric clinic. The front desk staff have been critical to our ability to deliver screening tools to caregivers, and thus, have benefited from education about the purpose of these tools, how to answer caregivers' questions, and other issues relevant to that first point of entry. Nursing staff often help caregivers to complete the screening tools, alert HSS when their patients have arrived, and might even refer families to HS based on concerns observed. Finally pediatric providers, although commonly very supportive of HS, may find it unusual to share a well-child visit with another professional, and may be surprised to learn that their previous developmental assessments may have been insufficient, due to a lack of attention to social emotional issues.

Nevertheless, the primary care setting remains a medical practice first and foremost; thus, the HS program must exist in a way that is mindful of the flow of the practice, the demands on the providers, and the metrics upon which that practice is measured, from productivity to compliance. We had to learn to speak the language of the practice, with regard to scheduling, documenting, and billing, and the standards for patient care— while skillfully adding in our own voices in measured and strategic ways.

Lesson #2: Documentation, Privacy, and Communication with Providers

Psychologists coming from traditional mental health clinics approach issues of documentation and communication in specific ways, many of which differ from those conventionally used in pediatrics. Throughout our years in an integrated set-ting, we have addressed multiple challenges and miscommunications that have arisen as a result. One of the earliest and most critical questions that arose was the extent to which HSS should include caregivers' personal details within their children's medical charts. For example, when HSSs conduct an intake interview, they always assess caregiver trauma history. After all, we—as mental health pro-fessionals—know the large impact that a parent's past trauma can have on their parenting style, and, thus, on a child's development. That said, we have grappled with the extent to which knowledge of a caregiver's trauma history is helpful or even necessary for the child's pediatrician. Patient privacy concerns require us to consider whether the HSS needs to obtain consent before communicating this information to the pediatrician, and if the information is included in the child's chart, the level of detail must also be considered.

As pioneers of this model, we have confronted these—among many other—ques-tions repeatedly. Questions of privacy, of which provider is entitled to what informa-tion, and of how best to document and communicate about sensitive issues are paramount to our practice. Not surprisingly, given the high level of complexity of these matters, we have not come to any sweeping conclusions. Rather, we have often opted to address these concerns on a case-by-case basis, seeking out consultation from each other and from experts in our field regarding regarding privacy and compliance. To date, our guiding principle has been to communicate to pediatricians only informa-tion deemed directly relevant to the child's care, and to do so with the minimal level of detail necessary (e.g., "mother has a long and severe trauma history," vs. details of said history). We inform caregivers that this is the manner in which we need to operate as a clinical team attempting to treat the whole family, including intergenerational dynamics and patterns. We have also attempted to provide ongoing education about these issues to clinic staff, so that we can continue to work together to serve our patients in the most respectful, legal, and ethical way possible.

This latter point is best illustrated by an example. During one well-child visit, a pediatrician unintentionally breached confidentiality by asking a mother about her experience with PMH therapy in front of her husband, who did not know that mother had been seeing a therapist through the HS program. In fact, this mother had sought therapy in order to process her discovery that her husband was having an affair, and she was worried he might find out that (a) she had this newfound knowledge, and (b) she had shared it with a professional. The therapist had not informed the pediatrician of the content of the therapy sessions, due to privacy regulations, as well as team consensus that the issues were not directly relevant to the child's care. However, she also had not let the pediatrician know that the mother's mere attendance was confidential; having been trained in multiple mental health settings, at which this is standard operating procedure, it did not occur to the PMH therapist that such a discussion was necessary. Following this incident, the HS staff made a point of educating the entire clinic staff about the importance of not mentioning a caregiver's therapy involvement unless he or she brings up the topic first; this is a very different approach for pediatricians, who are accustomed to following up with patient referrals as part of their job (e.g., "Have you been able to schedule an appointment with the cardiologist?").

Lesson #3: Isolation

The HS staff are often the only mental health providers within their pediatric clinics, and their feelings of isolation take many forms. On a purely practical level, there may not be a clear place within the administrative infrastructure to ensure that needs are met. Large medical practices function with clearly delineated roles, usually based on discipline (doctors, nurses, etc.), and HSSs not neatly fall within one of those spheres. Thus, tasks from identifying someone to cancel HS patients if one of the specialists is out sick to ensuring that HSSs become trained on the new billing system may become needlessly difficult. On a more personal level, it may be challenging to be the only mental health provider within a system of physical health. This difficulty may rear its head following a particularly intense clinical session, when there is no like-minded colleague with whom to debrief, but there may also be frustrations in explaining the nature of one's work in order to meet the standards of best practice. As one PMH therapist was stationed in an exam room with the asthma treatment equipment, it required multiple explanations to convey that constant interruptions during her clinical sessions were more than minor inconveniences, and may have actually been damaging to the goals at hand. The demanding nature of the work requires opportunities for ongoing supervision and collaboration, and it is necessary to create these systems within the pediatric care structure.

Conclusion

We do not pretend to have all of these issues figured out; we have remained humble, and continue to tweak and refine our program even today. That said, we believe the lessons we have learned—and, frankly, mistakes we have made—may save those creating their own early childhood integrated care programs valuable time and energy, and it is in that spirit we have shared them here.

Acknowledgements Funding for Healthy Steps at Montefiore has been provided by the Altman Foundation, The Price Family Foundation, The Tiger Foundation, The Marks Family Foundation, the Child Welfare Foundation, The Stavros Niarchos Foundation, The Grinberg Family Foundation, The Hearst Foundation, and the New York City Council Children's Mental Health under 5 Initiative. The authors also wish to thank Dr. Andrew Racine for leadership, support and guidance throughout the lifespan of Healthy Steps at Montefiore.

References

American Academy of Pediatrics. (2008). *Recommendations for preventative pediatric health care*. Elk Grove Village, IL: Author.

Briggs, R. A., Stettler, E. M., Silver, E. J., Schrag, R. D. A, Nayak, M., Chinitz, S., & Racine, A. D. (2012), Social emotional screening for infants and toddlers in primary care. *Pediatrics, 129(2)*, 1–8.

Felitti, V. J., Anda, R. F., Nordenberg, D., Williamson, D. F., Spitz, A. M., Edwards, V., … Marks, J. S. (1998). Relationship of childhood abuse and household dysfunction to many of the leading causes of death in adults. The Adverse Childhood Experiences (ACE) Study. *American Journal of Preventative Medicine, 14*, 245–258.

Jellinek, M. S., Murphy, J. M., Robinson, J., Feins, A., Lamb, S., & Fenton, T. (1988). Pediatric symptom checklist: Screening school-age children for psychosocial dysfunction. *The Journal of Pediatrics, 112*, 201–209.

Murphy, A., Steele, M., Dube, S. R., Bate, J., Bonuck, K., Meissner, P., … Steele, H. (2013). Adverse childhood experiences (ACEs) questionnaire and adult attachment interview (AAI): Implications for parent child relationships. *Child Abuse & Neglect, 38*(2), 224–233.

Chapter 8
Cultural Considerations in Integrated Early Childhood Behavioral Health

Helena Duch, Kate Cuno, and Miguelina Germán

Abstract Parenting practices of young children are influenced, in part, by a family's cultural and ethnic heritage. The rapidly changing and diverse population of families in the United States calls for integrated early childhood specialists to be sensitive and aware of the needs of these families. This chapter explores cultural differences in the context of three common referrals in early childhood, which include helping parents navigate behavior problems, feeding/nutrition issues, and sleeping difficulties. Using examples from research and real-life clinical scenarios, this chapter highlights how integrated early childhood specialists can be mindful of cultural influences on parenting practices in their work with families of diverse backgrounds, and describes clinical strategies to help establish strong bonds with culturally diverse families. Lastly, this chapter highlights the importance of being aware of one's own personal biases and opinions when helping parents incorporate evidence-based parenting techniques in a culturally informed and respectful way.

Keywords Culture • Cultural competence

Parenting practices are undeniably rooted in a family's culture. While there is a recognition of universal parenting goals across cultures (e.g., providing safe environments for children, conveying social norms), parents accomplish these goals in the context of cultural beliefs and varying economic and social circumstances (García Coll et al., 1996). When a family accesses primary care, these differences in cultural and socioeconomic contexts may come into play and impact the relationship with the provider, and ultimately the child's care.

H. Duch, Psy.D. (✉)
Columbia University, Mailman School of Public Health, New York, NY, USA
e-mail: hd90@columbia.edu

K. Cuno, Psy.D. • M. Germán, Ph.D.
Montefiore Health System, Bronx, NY, USA
e-mail: kcuno@montefiore.org; mgerman@montefiore.org

© Springer International Publishing Switzerland 2016   117
R.D. Briggs (ed.), *Integrated Early Childhood Behavioral Health
in Primary Care*, DOI 10.1007/978-3-319-31815-8_8

The child population in the United States has been changing rapidly in the last 15 years. In 1990, 69 % of the child population was White, 15 % African-American, 12 % Latino, 3 % Asian and Pacific Islander, and 1 % American Indian (The Annie E. Casey Foundation, 2014). By 2012, the population of Latino children doubled (24 %), and White children accounted for 53 % of the overall child population. These demographics reflect a rapidly changing and more diverse population, which calls for a workforce trained to be sensitive and responsive to the needs of diverse families (American Academy of Pediatrics, 2004; The Annie E. Casey Foundation, 2014).

The American Academy of Pediatrics (AAP) defines culturally effective pediatric healthcare as "the delivery of care within the context of appropriate physician knowledge, understanding, and appreciation of all cultural distinctions leading to optimal health outcomes" (American Academy of Pediatrics, 2004). Furthermore, the AAP advocates for culturally effective **care** versus **competence**, highlighting care as requiring knowledge, skills and demonstration of behaviors and attitudes that are responsive to cultural variability amongst patients and families (American Academy of Pediatrics, 2004). While competence refers to an individual's knowledge and skill, care goes beyond that to the actual practice and implementation of these skills to best meet the needs of families.[1]

As the pediatric population diversifies, the potential disconnect among patients, their families, and pediatric providers (who are still predominantly from a European majority culture) widens, and may pose challenges for families accessing and engaging with the healthcare system.

Differences in cultural attributes between providers and families that may impact clinical interactions may stem from differences in gender, sexual orientation, race, ethnicity, and socioeconomic status. In this chapter, we will focus on cultural considerations when working with families of racial/ethnic groups different from the European American ethnic majority in the USA. The chapter is not intended to be an exhaustive review of cultural differences in the early childhood period. Rather, we summarize existing literature as it relates to three common referrals to early childhood pediatric specialists: (1) behavior problems; (2) feeding/nutrition; and (3) sleeping.

Despite our focus on describing broad group differences, we acknowledge significant within-group variability amongst all groups (e.g., within and between countries of origin). We are limited in this chapter, and largely based on available research, to capture the rich variability that exists within groups and advocate for further research that combines different methodologies to describe nuanced culturally centered parenting practices. We also acknowledge that the literature has largely focused on a deficit model, highlighting areas of weakness for minority groups. We advocate for further research that describes the strengths of different culture groups as they promote child well-being.

---

[1] The AAP has developed a tool kit to help pediatric practitioners with providing culturally effective care: www.aap.org/en-us/professional-resources/practice-support/Patient-Management/pages/Culturally-Effective-Care-Toolkit-What-Is-Culturally-Effective-Pediatric-Care-.aspx.

Beyond their culture of origin, families' acculturation processes (changes in language, tradition, and values as a result of exposure to a new culture) also inform their parenting. When available, we discuss the impact of acculturation on feeding, sleep, and behavior.

Access to Pediatric Care

The State Children's Health Insurance Program and Medicaid expansions have made significant strides in extending health coverage to all children (The Annie E. Casey Foundation, 2014). Despite this success, ethnic and racial differences still exist in the number of children who have health insurance. While nationally about 7 % of children (about 5.3 million) remain uninsured, the numbers are close to double for American Indians (16 %) and Hispanic children (12 %) (The Annie E. Casey Foundation, 2014). In addition, perceptions of primary care quality seem to be impacted by a family's background, language and whether the family has a consistent source of care (Seid, Stevens, & Varni, 2003). Issues of access to care should be at the forefront for pediatric providers, as they ensure that all families in their community feel welcome and have the knowledge and resources to get consistent and high quality healthcare.

Discipline in Early Childhood: Working with Culturally Diverse Families

The question of how best to discipline young children is one that engenders much debate across the United States. A large survey study conducted in pediatric practices in 32 states and Puerto Rico found that the four most common discipline practices parents reported using with children aged 2–11 years were time out (45.2 %), removal of privileges (41.5 %), yelling (13.0 %), and spanking (8.5 %) (Barkin, Scheindlin, Ip, Richardson, & Finch, 2007). Among young children aged 2–5 years, parents were 25 % more likely to use both time out and spanking compared to older children. In this study, ethnic differences were reported with African-American parents endorsing higher rates of spanking and lower rates of time out compared to White parents. In addition, Spanish-speaking, Latino parents used time out and removal of privileges less than White parents. However, English-speaking, Latino parents used spanking and yelling *less* than White parents (Barkin et al., 2007). For integrated early childhood behavioral health practitioners who are often tasked with providing consultation to parents of young children with behavior problems, knowledge of differences in discipline practices among ethnic groups should inform their daily interactions with culturally diverse families.

Differences in behavior management practices may be interpreted through two common lenses: a sociocultural perspective which emphasizes macro-level knowledge of different cultural groups and a social cognition perspective which suggests clinicians examine individual-level and environment-specific influences in parenting. The sociocultural perspective suggests clinicians be alert and knowledgeable about cultural ideologies (i.e., values). For example, cultural groups vary to the extent they value autonomy versus interdependence (Johnson, Radesky, & Zuckerman, 2013; Suizzo, 2007; Tsai, Telzer, Gonzales, & Fuligni, 2015) and have varying beliefs about affective control (e.g., more acceptable for girls to cry than boys). A parent's interpretation of a young child's behavior can be influenced by cultural values. For example, a young child who repeatedly asks for something from a parent could be perceived as "talking back" (violating the value of *respeto* among traditional Latino families) or "negotiating" (congruent with the value of developing independence in the USA). Thus, cultural values may actually impact how a parent or early childhood behavioral health practitioner interprets a child's behavior. A social cognition perspective suggests that parenting goals, previous modeling (i.e., how parents were disciplined as children), and parental beliefs about age appropriate child development or competencies also influence the discipline strategies they choose (Miller, 1988; Ren & Pope Edwards, 2015).

A typical referral to an integrated early childhood behavioral health practitioner may involve a toddler or preschooler who is "acting out" or having "behavior problems." When consulting with these parents, it is often easy for clinicians to elicit parental goals for their young children. For example, typical parental goals may be that they want their child to "listen" more, do what he/she is told, and tantrum less. To address these concerns, numerous evidence-based interventions with parents suggest the following strategies: planned ignoring, positive attention, time out, and child-directed play (e.g., one-on-one time) (Eyberg et al., 2001; Patterson, 1979; Webster-Stratton, Rinaldi, & Reid, 2011). For example, the Incredible Years parenting program, which targets these skills, was found to be effective in addressing oppositional behaviors in a randomized controlled trial with low-income, Caucasian, African-American, Hispanic, and Asian mothers of young children (Reid, Webster-Stratton, & Beauchaine, 2001).

However, if early childhood behavioral health practitioners begin to teach these strategies after having elicited parental goals, but before conducting a more thorough and nuanced assessment of parental values, parents may ultimately not implement these suggested techniques due to an incongruence of the parenting recommendations with their value system. For example, while a parent may readily verbalize "I want my child to listen more and tantrum less," it may be more difficult to get a parent to identify the values and norms that shape how he or she feels about various discipline strategies. For example, parents from culturally diverse backgrounds may feel less comfortable admitting to a clinician that time out is considered an "American style" of parenting (Kim & Hong, 2007) that is not highly valued in their family.

A useful framework to help early childhood specialists conceptualize these consultations with culturally diverse families is the "Iceberg Model of Culture" (Hall, 1976). This model (also referred to as the onion model and the pyramid model) discusses the importance of the observable (e.g., race, social class, gender) and less visible aspects of cultures (preferences, implicit attitudes, beliefs, values) that influence the cultural context at large. This model's utility has been discussed by researchers within the healthcare setting (Flynn, Cooper, & Gary-Webb, 2013). Clinicians will be more effective in motivating parents to implement their suggested discipline techniques if they can elicit both the surface and deeper levels of communications (hence, the iceberg or onion metaphor). In this section, we describe some common discipline techniques and provide examples to help practitioners understand the challenges they may pose to parents of different cultural backgrounds.

Planned Ignoring

As a form of extinction, planned ignoring aims to weaken, decrease, or eliminate an unwanted behavior (Scheuermann & Hall, 2008). This discipline technique withholds reinforcement and signals to a child that inappropriate behavior will not lead to desired outcomes (Gable, Hester, Rock, & Hughes, 2009). Parents who come from cultures which place a high value on children being well behaved in public may have a difficult time when being told to ignore their children's misbehavior, particularly in settings outside the home or in front of extended family members. Calzada (2010) found in a study of Dominican and Mexican immigrant mothers living in the USA that the value of *respeto* had a greater emphasis on obedience/conformity than the US concept of respect and that mothers described deference, decorum, and behaving well in public as behavioral manifestations of *respeto*. She suggested that Latino parents who strongly endorse the *respeto* value may disagree or have difficulty implementing planned ignoring of behaviors such as making a face, name calling, or talking back (Calzada, 2010).

Positive Reinforcement

Parents can utilize verbal praise and other displays of positive attention to reinforce and maintain a desirable target behavior in a child (Alber & Heward, 2000). Research has found that positive attention provides a strong incentive for a child to retain newly learned skills and cooperate with peers and caretakers (Dishion & Patterson, 1996). Researchers who study parenting from culturally diverse groups such as Kim and Hong (2007) found that in a study with first-generation Korean parents in the USA, a common belief was that "American parents over used praising and showing affection" (p. 5) to their children. Other researchers have noted that among Korean families, warmth is often expressed nonverbally (Choi, Kim, Kim, & Park, 2013). In a study examining similarities and differences in mothers' parenting of preschoolers in China and the United States (Wu et al., 2002), Chinese mothers scored lower than US mothers on warmth/acceptance items, which included items asking about giving praise and verbalizing appreciation. A study by Horn et al. (2004) highlights the important role that socioeconomic status (SES) can play in within-group variability; they studied African-American parents of varying SES with children ages 1–3 years, and found that middle/upper SES African-American parents were significantly more likely to reward their child for positive behaviors compared to their lower SES counterparts.

Time Out

Time out is a behavior modification procedure that places a child in an environment of limited sensory stimulation in order to decrease the frequency of an undesirable and deviant target behavior (Fabiano et al., 2004; Wolf, McLaughlin, & Williams, 2006). A study of Puerto Rican families with children aged 4–6 years found that time out procedures in an empirically validated child behavior management intervention needed to be modified for this population (Matos, Torres, Santiago, Jurado, & Rodriguez, 2006). Specifically, children who actively refused to go to the time out chair or room were triggering the use of excessive force by the parents. Thus, the researchers proposed another procedure (e.g., loss of privileges) as an alternate discipline technique.

In our clinical experience, another barrier to the successful implementation of time out can be the opinion of extended family members, particularly when grandparents live with parents and their children. In primary care clinics in the Bronx, New York, parents from Latino or Caribbean/West Indian backgrounds have reported that their own parents criticize them or interfere when they try to implement time out at home with their children. Offering to meet with grandparents directly to discuss their concerns can help to increase their commitment to trying different techniques and ease tensions at home. The "adult" parents often share that it would be disrespectful to tell their own parents how to behave toward their grandchildren, and they welcome help getting all the caregivers on the same page.

Child-Directed Play (One-on-One Time)

Play offers an opportunity for parents to engage with their children (Ginsburg, 2007), and evidence shows that engaging in child-directed play increases children's compliance (Schuhmann, Foote, Eyberg, Boggs, & Algina, 1998). In general, most parents, regardless of their cultural background, can find it confusing to be told to play with their child as a way to increase their compliance. If the parent conceptualizes playing with the child as a reward to the child, being advised by an early childhood specialist to engage in play with a child who has engaged in noncompliant behavior can feel "wrong" to the parent in a way that violates their common sense. One evidence-based therapy that incorporates child-directed play is Parent–Child Interaction

Therapy (PCIT). McCabe, Yeh, Garland, Lau, and Chavez (2005) developed a version of PCIT that was culturally adapted for Mexican-American families (McCabe et al., 2005). They changed the name of the program to "Guiando a Niños Activos (GANAS)" (i.e., Guiding Active Children) and translated the Child-Directed Interaction component as "Ejercicios de Communicación," which in English translates as "Communication Exercises." The authors explained they had conducted focus groups with Mexican-American parents who indicated that seeking counseling services for their children carried much stigma. Thus, the program developers changed the names of the program and its components in an effort to destigmatize the techniques. They chose names that were congruent with the parents' viewpoints that improving parent–child communication was important. In a study with Mexican-American families with children ages 3–7 years, three conditions were compared: (1) the culturally modified version of PCIT discussed above called GANAS; (2) the original PCIT program; and (3) treatment as usual (TAU). Over the long term (6–24 months post treatment), GANAS significantly outperformed PCIT and TAU on a measure assessing child somatic, depressive, and anxiety symptoms (McCabe, Yeh, Lau, & Argote, 2012).

Physical Discipline

Few topics in parenting are more controversial than the use of physical discipline. Kazdin and Benjet (2003) outlined three views on spanking which are reflected among researchers, clinicians, and parents in most societies (Kazdin & Benjet, 2003). There is the pro-physical punishment perspective, the anti-physical punishment perspective, and the conditional physical punishment perspective. While the use of corporal punishment is not supported by the American Academy of Child and Adolescent Psychiatry (American Academy of Child & Adolescent Psychiatry, 2012; Committee on Psychosocial Aspects of Child and Family Health, 1998), a number of parents use this technique, particularly with young children (Barkin et al., 2007). Numerous studies have found negative outcomes associated with physical discipline of children such as increased aggression, delinquent behavior, lower internalization of parental morals/values, and poor parent–child relationship quality (Gershoff, 2002; MacKenzie, Nicklas, Brooks-Gunn, & Waldfogel, 2015). There is some evidence that the effects of physical discipline may differ for children from various cultural and socioeconomic backgrounds. For example, among African-American families, a number of studies have found no associations between physical discipline and externalizing behaviors if the overall parent–child relationship is high in warmth (Deater-Deckard, Dodge, Bates, & Pettit, 1996; Deater-Deckard, Ivy, & Petrill, 2006; McLoyd & Smith, 2002).

Many of the parents from culturally diverse backgrounds report they were spanked and physically disciplined in other ways when they were children (Marti, Snow, Wu, & Duch, 2015). When working with these families, early childhood behavioral specialists need to balance multiple goals including educating parents about the laws in their state regarding the use of physical discipline, assessing parents' opinions on the use of physical discipline, always ensuring child safety and well-being, and using motivational interviewing techniques in an attempt to increase parents' commitment to using other discipline techniques.

Discipline Conclusions and Practical Recommendations

Parents with young children who are having difficulty following rules at home or at day care/preschool often end up visiting early childhood behavioral specialists to seek assistance. These consultations represent an opportunity to help the parent–child dyad "reset" their interactions around these challenging moments of frustration in the parent–child relationship. Below we outline some general recommendations on how to approach consultations with families of diverse cultural backgrounds regarding the topic of discipline.

1. *Assess which discipline strategies were used in a parent's own childhood.* While using techniques to build rapport, ask the parents how they were disciplined when they were young children. Avoid expressing opinions or engaging in psychoeducation at this stage of the consultation.
2. *Assess and validate the parent's underlying goals, concerns, and values driving their current discipline strategies.* Making statements that help the parents believe you understand and respect their values is essential, such as "Of course you worry about raising a child who doesn't listen, especially in a neighborhood with lots of car traffic." Or, "It sounds like having a child that obeys quickly is very important to you." One subtle point for early childhood behavioral specialists is to validate the underlying parental goal or concern without expressing support for discipline techniques that the specialist wants to discourage (e.g., coercive discipline techniques).
3. *Combine continual assessment and validation.* Highlight the parent's feelings of frustration with the current situation. Weave the past and present together through your questioning. "What do you think was good about the way you were disciplined? Why do you think it may not be working with your child the way it worked for you?"
4. *While adopting a collaborative, respectful tone, it can help to motivate parents to try new techniques by highlighting the parent's freedom to choose and the lack of success of current alternatives.* For example, "It does not seem from what you've shared with me today that your current discipline strategies are working, is that right? Well, you can keep disciplining the way you have—you're in charge at home—and, I do have some other ideas about ways to discipline that I think could potentially help."
5. *Introduce new strategies.* Prior to introducing new strategies, be mindful of which discipline techniques you want to recommend as they may not match with the family's cultural values and practices. If you suspect the discipline practice

is culturally incongruent with the family's own values/practices, a helpful strategy would be to use humor to introduce a new technique. For example, you might introduce time out by saying, "This might feel very silly to you but…", which helps to foster a collaborative tone.

Nutrition and Feeding Practices: Working with Diverse Families

There are few things more important to new parents and caregivers than what and how much their children are eating. Baby and toddler nutrition and feeding are some of the most common pediatric consults in the early childhood years. There is wide variability in nutrition and feeding practices across and within cultural groups, and these practices sometimes align or may be in direct opposition to best practice recommendations from the AAP. Behavioral health practitioners are advised to explore families' feeding and diet customs without judgment, to understand the driver behind certain practices, and to assess how best to support families to enhance child well-being within a family's culture. Furthermore, feeding practices are intimately related to the availability of certain foods and the resources to access them, as well as cultural preferences for certain types of foods and cooking practices. Behavioral health practitioners should consider these issues when assessing nutrition and making recommendations to families.

We review broad similarities and differences amongst ethnic and racial groups in breastfeeding, introduction of solid foods, consumption of healthy and unhealthy foods, and general feeding practices.

Breastfeeding The AAP recommends exclusive breastfeeding for the first 6 months of an infant's life, followed by breastfeeding until age 12 months, as complementary foods are introduced (American Academy of Pediatrics, 2012). Thanks to significant public health efforts and campaigns that highlight the benefits of breastfeeding, rates have seen an overall increase in the last decade (Centers for Disease Control and Prevention, 2013). Despite these encouraging trends, differences exist amongst the percentage of children who were ever breastfed: Hispanic children have the highest prevalence of breastfeeding initiation of all ethnic groups (80 %), followed by Whites (75.2 %) and Blacks (58.9 %) (Centers for Disease Control and Prevention, 2013).

Disparities in breastfeeding initiation are also present for low-income and teenage mothers; those in the Special Nutrition Program for Women, Infants and Children (WIC) have an initiation rate of 67.5 % compared to 84.6 % of mothers in a higher income bracket, not eligible for WIC (Li, Darling, Maurice, Barker, & Grummer-Strawn, 2005). Similarly, younger mothers (under 20 years) have lower initiation rates (59.7 %) than those older than 30 years (79.3 %) (American Academy of Pediatrics, 2012; Li, Darling, Maurice, Barker, & Grummer-Strawn, 2005). Low maternal education and unmarried status are also associated with lower rates of breastfeeding (Centers for Disease Control and Prevention, 2013).

While many factors explain these disparities, most are not well understood. Access to healthcare that is supportive of breastfeeding is an important consideration. A recent study linked the Maternity Practices in Infant Nutrition and Care (MPINC) survey to US Census data on the percentage of Blacks living within a particular zip code for each health facility. The study concluded that facilities in zip code areas with higher percentages of Black residents were less likely to meet indicators for recommended practices supportive of breastfeeding (Lind, Perrine, Li, Scanlon, & Grummer-Strawn, 2014). Other studies have suggested that Black women are more likely to encounter unsupportive work environments and cultural norms that do not encourage initiation or duration of breastfeeding (American Academy of Pediatrics, 2012). Ethnographic studies with African-American mothers have identified reluctance to breastfeed in public, particularly for women living in inner-city neighborhoods with high population densities (Reeves & Woods-Giscombé, 2014). Home overcrowding and lack of privacy are also reported as factors that undermine breastfeeding, and additional common concerns relate to the perception that breast milk alone does not provide sufficient nutrition for the infant (Reeves & Woods-Giscombé, 2014).

On the Ground Example

In the pediatrician's office, many new moms will report pressure to breastfeed and shame around not breastfeeding. For instance, a young African-American mother, 22-years-old, was seen in a joint-visit by a pediatrician and a child psychologist for a regular well-child visit for her 4-month-old daughter. She reported that she had stopped producing breast milk around 2 months prior but was afraid to tell her child's pediatrician out of embarrassment and shame around "not being a good enough mother to feed her child." This particular mother was unaware of the supply and demand function of breast milk production and unfortunately, had she told her pediatrician about her limited supply early on, her feelings of shame and embarrassment, as well as the loss of the beneficial nutrition to her daughter and building of the parent–child bond, could have been avoided.

Fathers or spouses play an important role in supporting breastfeeding as well. Women who have supportive partners and extended family are more likely to initiate and sustain breastfeeding than those who do not have supportive networks (Reeves & Woods-Giscombé, 2014).

Acculturation also plays a role in breastfeeding. Initiation, duration, and exclusive breastfeeding are more likely in less acculturated Hispanic mothers than in more acculturated ones (Gibson, Diaz, Mainous, & Geesey, 2005).

Little is known about breastfeeding initiation and duration for other ethnic groups. No current national prevalence is available for Asian-Americans or Native Americans, and the research relies on relatively small studies. The rate of ever breastfeeding amongst Asian-Americans is approximately 75 %, however duration is short and by 6 months, the rates are estimated to be lower than for Hispanics and Whites (County of Los Angeles Department of Health, 2004; Lee, 2013). Some cultural practices may contribute to this trend. One example in the Chinese American community is the practice of *Zuo Yuezi*, where the mother is encouraged to stay home and refrain from going outdoors for a period of time after birth in order to bond with her newborn. The practice of Zuo Yuezi has been described in the literature as both protective of breastfeeding and a risk to breastfeeding (Lee, 2013; Lee & Brann, 2014). Reportedly, during this time, mothers receive significant pressure from extended family members discouraging them from breastfeeding and encouraging early introduction of solids (Lee & Brann, 2014). Other practices such as sending infants back to China to be raised by grandparents or extended family while parents work in the United States are also identified as risks (Lee & Brann, 2014).

Breastfeeding in Native American families is significantly understudied. The few data points that do exist point to an estimated 13 % of American Indian families who exclusively breastfed their infants for 6 months (Eckhardt et al., 2014). Survey research has highlighted American Indian women's knowledge of the importance of exclusive breastfeeding but reports less information around the benefits of breastfeeding for preventing disease and promoting positive development (Eckhardt et al., 2014).

Understanding cultural norms, access and support for breastfeeding are essential in promoting positive practices. Providers should examine their facilities' breastfeeding supportive practices and routinely discuss families' beliefs, supports, and barriers as they relate to breastfeeding initiation and maintenance.

Introduction of solid foods A national study using the 2000 National Survey of Early Childhood Health found that race and ethnic differences in the introduction of solids depend on maternal education (Kuo, Inkelas, Slusser, Maidenberg, & Halfon, 2011). Overall, mothers with less than high school education are more likely to introduce solids before the recommended 4–6 month window; however, there are cultural differences within this group, such that Whites are more likely to introduce solids early and Blacks late (Kuo et al., 2011). Survey research with American Indian mothers concluded that about 50 % introduced infant cereals in the bottle before 4–6 months (Eckhardt et al., 2014). Early introduction of solid foods (before the age of 4–6 months) has been associated, especially amongst formula-fed babies, with higher rates of childhood obesity (Huh, Rifas-Shiman, Taveras, Oken, & Gillman, 2011).

The presence of elders may play a role in the timing of solid food introduction. Grandparents have been reported to promote introduction of solids early in an infant's life. Ethnographic work with Black teenage moms and Chinese American moms both point to the important role that grandparents and extended family members have in determining when and what an infant is fed (Lee & Brann, 2014; Bentley, Gavin, Black, & Teti, 1999). Behavioral health practitioners should assess the family composition of pediatric patients and explore the role that extended family plays in infant feeding.

Early feeding practices associated with overweight and obesity in childhood
Obesity in early childhood has a national prevalence of 8.4 %; however, the rates are almost double for children from low socioeconomic backgrounds (15 %) (Ogden, Carroll, Kit, & Flegal, 2014). In addition to the early introduction of solid foods noted above, several other early feeding practices have been linked to the development of overweight and obesity in childhood.

In a large national randomized study designed to prevent obesity, when assessed at child age 2 months, about 10 % of families had introduced solid foods, almost half put infants in bed with bottles, and many propped bottles and always fed their infant as a way to soothe them when they are upset (Perrin et al., 2014). Remarkably, even at this young age group, 90 % of children were exposed to television and 66 % did not meet tummy time recommendations. Black and Hispanic parents reported more frequent use of these strategies, such as putting children to sleep with a bottle, bottle propping, encouraging children to finish all their milk and less tummy time (Perrin et al., 2014).

Other studies have identified early introduction of solids before 4 months, sleeping less than 12 h per day, drinking sugar-sweetened beverages, and rapid infant weight gain as risk factors more commonly associated with practices in Black and Hispanic families (Taveras, Gillman, Kleinman, Rich-Edwards, & Rifas-Shiman, 2010).

Feeding practices Certain feeding practices that aim to control children's feeding appear to be common amongst many of the most commonly studied ethnic/racial groups. Parental overcontrol of feeding has been associated with higher body mass index (BMI) (Cachelin, Thompson, & Phimphasone, 2014). Practices such as pressuring children to eat and incentivizing with bribes/rewards are reported amongst the majority of ethnic, racial groups, and across socioeconomic strata (Sherry et al., 2004). In a sample of African-American preschoolers, pressure to eat was associated with increased weight (Powers, Chamberlin, Schaick, Sherman, & Whitaker, 2006).

While more controlling feeding practices have been associated with higher BMIs in White and African-American children, the relationship appears to be inverse for Chinese American children, where more controlled feeding practices led to lower BMI outcomes (Cachelin et al., 2014). In one study, Chinese American parents who had an authoritarian or authoritative style had children with lower BMI than parents with an indulgent parenting style. Interestingly, as families became more acculturated, their parenting became more indulgent (Pai & Contento, 2014). Within Hispanic families, those less acculturated were more likely to push their children to eat, use foods to calm their children, and use positive incentives to get them to eat more (Evans et al., 2011).

On the Ground Example

The problematic consequences of parents being overly controlling about children's feeding are perhaps best illustrated by an example. A young mother of South Asian descent was referred to a behavioral health practitioner by the pediatrician as her nearly 4-year-old son was, by her report, an extremely picky eater and not interested in eating anything other than juice and candy. The provider met with the family and learned within the first visit that the household consisted of many families from multiple generations, many of whom had their own opinions on how much the child should and should not be eating. Specifically, the mother spoke at length about how, in the first year or two of her son's life, she felt significant pressure to continuously soothe him with food from her relatives who were easily disturbed by his age-appropriate crying. The child's mother noted that for the first 3 years of his life, she fed her son every 2–3 h and when he became mobile as a toddler, she continued to spend up to 2 h forcing him to eat solid food by feeding him herself, despite his ability to feed himself with his hands or a utensil. She noted frustration that he would be more interested in doing other things and would not sit still to eat for more than 15 min. The mother repeatedly stated that if she did not feed him, she knew "he would never eat," and she was incredibly fearful of her son being malnourished. This pattern of forcing food can spiral into a cycle in which the child loses his bodily cues for hunger and does not develop the self-awareness of satiation, as was the case in this particular example.

Income differences are also related to feeding practices. The use of food as reward is more common in low-income children than in their more affluent counterparts (Hendy & Williams, 2012), while picky eating, which is associated with lower dietary variety and less vegetable consumption, is more common in higher income families (Evans et al., 2011).

While an important area to assess, there is scarce research in the role of fathers in feeding. One systematic review of the literature on father feeding practices concludes that dads are more likely to use pressure to get their kids to eat, but are less likely to monitor their children's food intake and limit their access (Khandpur, Blaine, Fisher, & Davison, 2014).

Consumption of fruits and vegetables Across ethnic and racial groups, parents are motivated by similar desires to provide good nutrition for their children and avoid the overconsumption of unhealthy foods (e.g., sweets, processed foods) (Sherry et al., 2004). Nationally, there are few differences between race and ethnicity in the percentage of youth who consumed vegetables and fruits (Nielsen, Rossen, Harris, & Ogden, 2014). These few differences point to African-Americans reportedly consuming more fruit juice and starchy vegetables, while Hispanics consumed more vegetables than other groups (Nielsen et al., 2014).

While differences are not significant across ethnic/racial groups, SES seems to influence the kinds of foods that children have access to. Studies have identified that children from lower income backgrounds may have less daily consumption of fruits and vegetables and overall higher consumption of foods high in fats (Hendy & Williams, 2012).

Acculturation for several groups appears to have a negative effect on the consumption of fruits and vegetables. More acculturated Hispanic children consume fewer fruits and vegetables (Chaparro, Langellier, Wang, Koleilat, & Whaley, 2014), while more acculturated Chinese American families put less pressure on their children to eat healthy foods (Pai & Contento, 2014). The mechanisms by which acculturation affects diet are still largely unexplored and not understood.

Nutrition and Feeding Conclusions and practical applications Nutrition and feeding are primary concerns for families, regardless of their background. Across groups, families want the best nutritional outcomes for their children and share a concern to provide healthy food choices and limit unhealthy ones. Significant variability is present in early feeding practices, particularly around rates of breastfeeding initiation, duration, and introduction of solid foods.

Despite an overall commitment to positive nutrition, issues of access to resources, knowledge, attitudes, cultural values, and social supports hinder families' abilities to promote healthy habits. This may be particularly true for families residing with elder relatives, who might have conflicting opinions regarding the introduction of solid foods or initiation of breastfeeding.

Early childhood behavioral health providers should conduct a comprehensive assessment of families' feeding habits, considering the family's resources, social networks, access to services, lifestyle, and cultural values as they relate to breastfeeding, food choices, and feeding practices.

Sleep in Infancy and Early Childhood: A Cross-Cultural Perspective

Sleep patterns and practices are often a major source of concern for parents and healthcare professionals, especially in the first few years of life (Mindell, Sadeh, Kohyama, & How, 2010; Mindell, Sadeh, Kwon, & Goh, 2013; Mindell, Sadeh, Wiegand, How, & Goh, 2010). Sleep is determined by biological and cultural factors, and it is the interaction between these two factors that affects the establishment of developmental and behavioral norms, expectations, and perceptions surrounding infant sleep patterns (Mindell et al., 2013; Mindell, Sadeh, Kohyama, et al., 2010; Mindell, Sadeh, Wiegand, et al., 2010). The current research supports approaching infant sleep behaviors through a transactional model that emphasizes the ongoing bidirectional links between heavily culturally influenced parental factors (parenting practices, beliefs, expectations, and emotions) and the developmental milestones related to infant sleep (Sadeh, Tikotzky, & Scher, 2010).

Many aspects of sleep are influenced by cultural standards including how we sleep, with whom, and where. For example, several tribal societies across the globe encourage children to sleep when tired throughout the day, even when in the presence of others or during social gatherings (Jenni & O'Connor, 2005). Cultural norms also determine the boundaries between normal and problematic sleep behavior. That is, the cultural regulation of sleep patterns involves larger cultural values and social pressures, which may or may not be about sleep, including things such as social class and rank, gender roles, family structures and behaviors, religious practices and beliefs, and standards of morality for personal behavior (Jenni & O'Connor, 2005).

In this section, we review the cross-cultural literature on sleep behaviors, patterns, and problems of infants and young children, under the general understanding that sleep is a biologically driven behavior of any child that is strongly shaped and interpreted by cultural values and beliefs of the parents.

Sleep Characteristics and Patterns

Routines and schedules Cross-cultural research reveals that where and how parents put their children to sleep, and concerns parents have about their children's sleep can reveal valuable information about culturally embedded practices, values, and goals that shape the family context of child development (Milan, Snow, & Belay, 2007). Within the United States, physicians often recommend that parents maintain specific routines to facilitate children's sleep and numerous parenting books provide advice on how to achieve this goal. The importance placed on bedtime routines and continuity in the United States is consistent with the view that maintaining sleep schedules facilitates children's developing capacity for self-regulation (Milan et al., 2007). In contrast, bedtime routines do not play a prominent role in family life in countries where being "well-regulated" is less of an individual goal. In Italy, for example, children are more involved in familial activities during the evening and as a result, tend to fall asleep when and where they are tired (Milan et al., 2007; Jenni & O'Connor, 2005).

Additionally, self-reported rates of a regular bedtime routine are lower for African-American, Latino, and Asian families relative to White families (Crabtree et al., 2005; Milan et al., 2007; Mindell et al., 2013). White mothers are significantly more likely to report giving comfort objects as part of the bedtime routine compared with African-American families. Additionally, White families are more likely to report telling a bedtime story compared with African-American and Latino families. Other noted differences between groups include young children in Asian countries having later bedtimes, later wake times, and less nighttime sleep (Mindell et al., 2013; Mindell, Sadeh, Kohyama, et al., 2010; Mindell, Sadeh, Wiegand, et al., 2010).

Regarding specific aspects of bedtime routines, children from predominantly Caucasian backgrounds most often fall asleep independently in their own crib or bed after a bedtime routine including an after-dinner bath, dressing in a particular nightdress, telling stories and singing lullabies, holding, rocking, and nursing the child to sleep (Mindell, Sadeh, Kohyama, et al., 2010; Mindell, Sadeh, Wiegand, et al., 2010), putting the child to bed and then leaving the child alone in his or her room (Jenni & O'Connor,

On the Ground Example

Within a primary care setting in an area of the Bronx largely populated with families who have immigrated from India and Bangladesh, sleeping difficulties are among the top three reasons for which a pediatrician will refer a family to an early childhood behavioral health practitioner. This is perhaps best illustrated with an example. Earlier this year, a 3-year-old boy was referred to the clinic's early childhood behavioral health practitioner for not sleeping through the night and overall disrupted sleep. This particular boy and his mother were of Bengali descent and upon meeting them for the initial visit, the practitioner learned that the young boy had been sleeping in his mother's bed since he was born and did not nap independently either. While this boy's mother was frustrated by waking up frequently to her son crying, asking for food or water, or just needing attention, the notion that part of the solution to this problem would involve him sleeping elsewhere was shocking to her. Additionally, the practitioner had to consider the other members of the particular living circumstances. The recommendation to place the child into a bed in a separate room was not possible for this family who resided in a one-bedroom apartment with three children under 6 years of age. With sensitivity to the logistical constraints around recommending a traditional sleep training regime, the practitioner encouraged the boy's mother to practice having her son learn to self-soothe during the day by instituting a consistent nap time. After this was achieved and the boy began falling asleep without his mother being physically next to him, his mother began to see that this new sense of independence was not going to negatively impact his development nor the parent–child relationship. This mother became more confident in actively ignoring her son's bids for attention during the night, and allowing him the space and time to fall back asleep on his own.

2005). In Asian countries, however, parents are more likely to have children fall asleep with them in their bed, feed their children to sleep, and hold their children until they fall asleep (Mindell, Sadeh, Kohyama, et al., 2010; Mindell, Sadeh, Wiegand, et al., 2010).

Duration Studies suggest a wide range in sleep duration in young infants. Overall, calculations revealed a decline in sleep duration at approximately 10 min per month between 1 and 6 months of age, slowing to 5 min per month between 7 and 12 months. Cross-cultural analyses of this data revealed that sleep duration of children ages 0 through 12 months was shorter in predominantly Asian countries/regions compared to dominantly Caucasian/non-Asian countries by 1 h. These differences were related to later bedtimes rather than daytime sleep, and suggest a strong culturally based influence on nighttime sleep behaviors.

Some aspects of sleep appear more biologically based than cultural, and thus show less cross cultural variation. Overall, the average number of night wakings, duration of nocturnal wakefulness, and number of daytime naps decreases with age, and the last nap extends in duration, cross-culturally as well (Palmstierna, Sepa, &

Ludvigsson, 2008; Sadeh, Mindell, Luedtke, & Wiegand, 2009). However, while daytime sleep duration is mostly related to age, nocturnal sleep duration appears to be mostly explained by multiple ecological and contextual factors, with sleeping in a separate room being the strongest predictor (Sadeh et al., 2009).

On the Ground Example

A very common concern of new parents is how to help their child fall asleep without being breastfed. Across cultures, within the primary care clinic of the Bronx mentioned above, mothers are frequently referred to the early childhood behavioral health practitioner, frustrated, tired, and anxious to establish a bed-time routine that allows for more independence on their child's part. Thankfully, there are tried and true interventions that help with this problem, but they all stem from the principle of allowing the child to tolerate age appropriate levels of distress, and in turn, helping the mother to tolerate her child's distress. It is this particular practitioner's experience that Caucasian mothers are somewhat more receptive to this suggestion and when they abide by recommendations, report significant improvements within 5–7 days. However, more mothers from South Asia than of Caucasian descent within the above mentioned clinic have reported struggles with the "cry it out" method. On multiple occasions, mothers from an Asian cultural background have cited multiple reasons for their inability to be consistent with this method including pressure from extended family members and partners to attend to the child's perceived need for comfort. In their own words, they have described being told they are "not doing their jobs as mothers" if they allow their children to cry for extended periods of time at night. Let the reader be aware this is based on a few select cases within this particular location of the Bronx and may not represent the greater South Asian immigrant population. This particular practitioner has found the most helpful interventions in these situations are to involve all family members in the conversation, build their awareness of the mother's distress, and problem-solve within the families' value system and general expectations to find a schedule of weaning that is consistent with their particular ideals.

Nighttime waking Frequent nighttime waking is one of the most common sleep difficulties reported by parents of young children across cultures (Jenni & O'Connor, 2005). Number of nighttime wakings over the first 24 months of life shows a decline in frequency from 1 to 6 months and continued decline from 7 to 24 months, showing an overall inverse relationship with age across all cultures (Galland, Taylor, Elder, & Herbison, 2012). Some predictors of night waking include breastfeeding back to sleep, not sleeping in a separate room, giving a bottle during the night, bringing the child to the parents' bed, and an irregular bedtime routine (Sadeh et al., 2009).

Naps There is limited research on the subject of daytime napping and its relationship to both nighttime sleep patterns and sleep requirements as well as to cultural responses to various forms of daytime sleep for children. However, some researchers have begun to conceptualize these ideas based on "nap" cultures, in which individual or collective napping occurs and is considered normal but other aspects of social life continue versus "siesta" cultures, referring specifically to those societies in which nap or rest time at the midday is institutionalized to the extent that social and commercial life closes down for the duration (Jenni & O'Connor, 2005). Cultures that institutionalize napping are significantly different than American and Northern European sleep cultures, in which daytime sleep is discouraged and avoided except for infants and very young children.

Co-sleeping Versus Independent Sleeping

The norm for children in many parts of the world is to sleep with adults or siblings, if not in the same bed itself, at least the same room (Jenni & O'Connor, 2005; Latz, Wolf, & Lozoff, 1999; Morelli, Rogoff, Oppenheim, & Goldsmith, 1992). Moreover, less industrialized but highly technologically advanced communities practice co-sleeping. For instance, in Japan, infants are socialized to have increasingly interdependent relations with others whereas in America, the infant is increasingly encouraged to be independent of others (Jenni & O'Connor, 2005). American parents have explained their practice of separation as an effort to instill independence, whereas

On the Ground Example

In "reactive co-sleeping" families, one common reason for this behavior includes a toddler's response to a second child being born and his or her need to return to his or her parent's bed for comfort and a sense of inclusion. Another common occurrence is the negatively reinforcing behavior on the parent's part to include his or her child in the adult's bed in response to a bad dream, sickness, or fear on the child's part. For instance, a young mother and her 4-year-old daughter were referred to the early childhood behavioral health practitioner at the abovementioned clinic for help in getting the young girl to go back to sleeping in her own room. This particular family had recently moved out of their home where the mother was the victim of domestic violence. They were able to stay with a family member; however, since entering that home around 9 months prior, the young girl was scared to sleep independently. It was only during the intake that the practitioner learned of the past exposure to domestic violence and the mother's tendency to allow her daughter to sleep with her for safety purposes. Had this particular family not had access to behavioral health within the pediatrician's office, it is likely recommendations would have been given to retrain the child to sleep on her own without careful consideration of the emotional reasons maintaining the co-sleeping behavior. After careful consideration of this particular dyad's unique situation, and interventions to build the child's sense of safety in her new home, she began successfully sleeping in her own bed and room within 1 month.

non-Western cultures often emphasize the value of closeness and establishing the parent–child bond (Morelli et al., 1992). Additionally, American families cite reasons related to fear of establishing a habit that will be difficult to break, safety issues, and feeling uncomfortable with the idea of wanting their child in their bed in general.

Within the United States, the incidence of co-sleeping varies greatly and appears to be influenced by ethnicity. African-American families report the highest incidence of co-sleeping, followed by Hispanic families, with Caucasian families reporting the lowest incidence (Mao, Burnham, Goodlin-Jones, Gaylor, & Anders, 2004; Milan et al., 2007; Sadeh et al., 2010). Among Caucasian families, co-sleeping was associated with low SES (Mao et al., 2004; Sadeh et al., 2010) and education level (Wolf & Lozoff, 1989). Additionally, American Caucasian families tend to be "reactive co-sleepers," who co-sleep in reaction to a sleep problem, whereas African-American and Hispanic-American families tend to co-sleep because of cultural tradition (Medoff & Schaefer, 1993). Among "reactive co-sleeping" families, there is a documented association between co-sleeping and infant sleep problems including difficulty falling asleep and frequent nighttime waking.

Parental Perception of Sleep Problems

Parental beliefs and cultural preferences such as a high value placed on individual independence or on familial interdependence have been cited as "driving forces" for choosing sleep arrangements and interpreting children's sleep behaviors (Jenni & O'Connor, 2005). For example, in a recent study of children's sleep habits in the United States and China, Liu et al. (2005) found that Chinese children were reported to have many more sleep problems, including difficulty falling asleep and daytime sleepiness (Liu, Liu, Owens, & Kaplan, 2005). Similar results were found in the Latz et al. study in 1999, wherein both Japanese and American parents acknowledged that isolating a child at night was stressful but interpreted the experience differently (Latz et al., 1999). In the United States, solitary sleep is thought to engender independence and ensure privacy for parents, which supersede the child's perceived need. Japanese parents acknowledge the same developmental struggle with separation but in acceding to the child's need, emphasize the value of dependence as the primary socializing experience.

In addition to cultural differences in parental perception of sleep problems, research has indicated that distorted parental perception of children's sleep patterns has a negative outcome on child sleep problems themselves (Sadeh et al., 2010). For example, maternal cognitions focused on the possibility that infants are distressed when they awake at night, and therefore need parental help, predict and are more often associated with frequent nighttime waking, whereas cognitions emphasizing the importance of limiting parental nighttime involvement predict more consolidated sleep (Mindell, Sadeh, Kohyama, et al., 2010; Mindell, Sadeh, Wiegand, et al., 2010; Sadeh et al., 2010). Overall, mothers who put more emphasis on infant distress in their understanding of sleep problems and nighttime waking are more likely to be actively involved during bedtime and at night, and this particular type of involvement is associated with more disrupted sleep (Adair, Bauchner, Philipp, Levenson, & Zuckerman, 1991; Anders, Halpern, & Hua, 1992; Mindell, Sadeh, Kohyama, et al., 2010; Mindell, Sadeh, Wiegand, et al., 2010; Sadeh et al., 2010; Tikotzky & Sadeh, 2009). Sadeh et al. (2007) explored the notion that parents tend to have internal representations of their infants even prior to their birth which then shape the actual experience of the baby and his or her development (Sadeh, Flint-Ofir, Tirosh, & Tikotzky, 2007). They found that sleep problems in early childhood were largely associated with ambivalent feelings toward the child and a sense of incompetence as a parent. Therefore, most infant/toddler sleep interventions rely heavily on parents as the change agents, and focus specifically on the alteration of parental cognitions and behaviors to facilitate better infant sleep.

Sleep Conclusions and Practical Applications

Infant sleep problems are a major concern in the early years of a child's life and are often a source of family distress that can disrupt the well-being of parents and children. It is important that early childhood behavioral health providers deliver effective sleep interventions as research has shown that neurocognitive functioning can be influenced by sleep behavior in children (Crabtree et al., 2005; O'Brien & Gozal, 2004). Specifically, children who have disrupted sleep are more likely to manifest deficits in neurocognitive and behavioral functioning including learning, memory, and hyperactive behavior.

With the increasing diversity in the United States, there is a growing potential for early childhood professionals and families to have differing views on what is expected or desired regarding children's sleep, which can ultimately interfere with the health and well-being of the child. Early childhood professionals are responsible for recognizing the cultural environment in which children live and the manner by which cultural beliefs and values interact with the needs of the individual child and with biological aspects of his or her sleep patterns. Additionally, professionals have the responsibility to attend to their own cultures' values and preferences and to the ways in which they respond based on their own expectations. Overall, understanding early childhood sleep problems involves a thorough look at all parental factors that may be contributing to or maintaining sleep problems (e.g., culture, parental cognitions, psychopathology). Educating parents on realistic perceptions and expectations and on sleep promoting practices is a major strategy in resolving infant sleep problems.

Conclusions

We have presented significant similarities and differences in how families from diverse backgrounds approach young children's feeding, sleep and behavior. As stated in the introduction to this chapter, our review is in no way comprehensive of the rich diversity present in the United States, and particularly of intragroup differences. The research examining more nuanced differences within groups is very limited and often draws from small samples.

We have enumerated many factors that influence families' decision-making: access to resources, information, beliefs, cultural values, their own upbringing, education, social networks and SES, amongst many others. Early childhood behavioral healthcare practitioners are advised to pay close attention to how these issues relate to parenting, and routinely assess their impact in families' practices.

To conclude, we provide five general recommendations to early childhood specialists to ensure careful consideration of parenting differences within their practice, regardless of the families' background.

1. In order to establish strong, working relationships with families, we must above all listen to families' narratives, without judgment, to learn how and why they espouse certain practices. Victor Bersntein states "people do not listen until they feel heard." (Bernstein, 2002). Creating a culturally informed environment in which to have these conversations with families will provide a window into their points of view, and save the behavioral health practitioners time and misunderstanding in the long run.
2. In order to listen without judgment, one must be aware of their own beliefs and values as they relate to these issues. Professional organizations such as the AAP and the American Psychological Association advise practitioners to systematically examine their personal beliefs and assumptions (American Psychological Association, 2002). Self-awareness is paramount when working with families who hold different values from one's own.
3. As we seek to reconcile culturally disparate parenting practices, it may be helpful to distinguish between "unacceptable" versus "disagreeable" practices. An unacceptable practice is one that is against the law or that puts the child in danger, and must be addressed immediately. However, there are many practices that may be disagreeable to the provider but acceptable, and culturally preferable, to the family (Bernstein, 2002). Working with diverse families, we must assess unacceptable versus disagreeable and support families to make their own choices, even if they are not congruent with our own beliefs (Bernstein, 2002).
4. Beyond the individual practitioner, close attention also needs to be paid to the physical environment of the practice to ensure that it represents and is responsive to families. For example, it is important to examine pictures, brochures, and print materials to make sure they depict different races, genders, family compositions, language and literacy levels, relevant to the particular practice.
5. Bridging language barriers is difficult, particularly when the provider is not fluent in the families' language. The AAP offers recommendations on training and working with interpreters and using technology to address this gap (American Academy of Pediatrics, 2004). Practitioners need to pay close attention to verbal and nonverbal communication and how language barriers (and health literacy) may affect treatment and care.

It is apparent that over time, the cultural attributes of children and families, including race, ethnicity, language, gender, among others, will continue to be different from those of the individual practitioner. In turn, changing demographics have implications for the use of medical and behavioral health services as well as the effective delivery of interventions. Moreover, an ever-changing population requires sensitive attention from pediatricians and behavioral health practitioners nationwide. This review serves as a call to child healthcare providers to attend to the unique impact of cultural attributes on common parenting challenges in the first years of life.

References

Adair, R., Bauchner, H., Philipp, B., Levenson, S., & Zuckerman, B. (1991). Night waking during infancy: Role of parental presence at bedtime. *Pediatrics, 87*(4), 500–504.

Alber, S. R., & Heward, W. L. (2000). Teaching students to recruit positive attention: A review and recommendations. *Journal of Behavioral Education, 10*(4), 177–204.

American Academy of Child & Adolescent Psychiatry. (2012). *Policy statement on corporal punishment*. Retrieved from https://www.aacap.org/aacap/policy_statements/2012/Policy_Statement_on_Corporal_Punishment.aspx.

American Academy of Pediatrics. (2004). Ensuring culturally effective pediatric care: Implications for education and health policy. *Pediatrics, 114*(6), 1667–1685.

American Academy of Pediatrics. (2012). Policy statement breastfeeding and the use of human milk. *Pediatrics, 129*(3), e827–e841.

American Psychological Association. (2002). *Guidelines on multicultural education, training, research, practice, and organizational change for psychologists*. Washington, DC.

Anders, T. F., Halpern, L., & Hua, J. (1992). Sleeping through the night: A developmental perspective. *Pediatrics, 90*, 554–560.

Barkin, S., Scheindlin, B., Ip, E., Richardson, I., & Finch, S. (2007). Determinants of parental discipline practices: A national sample from primary care practices. *Clinical Pediatrics, 46*(1), 64–69.

Bentley, M., Gavin, L., Black, M., & Teti, L. (1999). Infant feeding practices of low-income, African-American, adolescent mothers: An ecological, multigenerational perspective. *Social Science & Medicine, 49*(8), 1085–1100.

Bernstein, V. (2002). Strengthening families through strengthening relationships: Supporting the parent-child relationship through home visiting. *Newsletter of Infant Mental Health Promotion Project (IMP), 35*, 1–5.

Cachelin, F. M., Thompson, D., & Phimphasone, P. (2014). Impact of Asian American mothers' feeding beliefs and practices on child obesity in a diverse community sample. *Asian American Journal of Psychology, 5*(3), 223.

Calzada, E. J. (2010). Bringing culture into parent training with Latinos. *Cognitive and Behavioral Practice, 17*(2), 167–175.

Centers for Disease Control and Prevention. (2013). Progress in increasing breastfeeding and reducing racial/ethnic differences—United States, 2000–2008 births. *MMWR. Morbidity and Mortality Weekly Report, 62*(5), 277–280.

Chaparro, M. P., Langellier, B. A., Wang, M. C., Koleilat, M., & Whaley, S. E. (2014). Effects of parental nativity and length of stay in the US on fruit and vegetable intake among WIC-enrolled preschool-aged children. *Journal of Immigrant and Minority Health*, 1–6.

Choi, Y., Kim, Y., Kim, S., & Park, I. (2013). Is Asian American parenting controlling and harsh? Empirical testing of relationships between Korean American and Western parenting measures. *Asian American Journal of Psychology, 4*(1), 19.

Committee on Psychosocial Aspects of Child and Family Health. (1998). Guidance for effective discipline. *Pediatrics, 101*(4), 723–728.

County of Los Angeles Department of Health. (2004). *Breastfeeding practices*. Los Angeles, CA: Los Angeles Department of Health.

Crabtree, V., Korhonen, J., Montgomery-Downs, H., Jones, V. F., O'Brien, L. M., & Gozal, D. (2005). Cultural influences on the bedtime behaviors of young children. *Sleep Medicine, 6*(4), 319–324.

Deater-Deckard, K., Dodge, K. A., Bates, J. E., & Pettit, G. S. (1996). Physical discipline among African American and European American mothers: Links to children's externalizing behaviors. *Developmental Psychology, 32*(6), 1065.

Deater-Deckard, K., Ivy, L., & Petrill, S. A. (2006). Maternal warmth moderates the link between physical punishment and child externalizing problems: A parent-offspring behavior genetic analysis. *Parenting: Science and Practice, 6*(1), 59–78.

Dishion, T. J., & Patterson, S. G. (1996). *Preventive parenting with love, encouragement, and limits: The preschool years*. Eugene, OR: Castalia.

Eckhardt, C. L., Lutz, T., Karanja, N., Jobe, J. B., Maupomé, G., & Ritenbaugh, C. (2014). Knowledge, attitudes, and beliefs that can influence infant feeding practices in American Indian Mothers. *Journal of the Academy of Nutrition and Dietetics, 114*(10), 1587–1593.

Evans, A., Seth, J. G., Smith, S., Harris, K. K., Loyo, J., Spaulding, C., … Gottlieb, N. (2011). Parental feeding practices and concerns related to child underweight, picky eating, and using food to calm differ according to ethnicity/race, acculturation, and income. *Maternal & Child Health Journal, 15*(7), 899–909. doi:10.1007/s10995-009-0526-6.

Eyberg, S. M., Funderburk, B. W., Hembree-Kigin, T. L., McNeil, C. B., Querido, J. G., & Hood, K. K. (2001). Parent-child interaction therapy with behavior problem children: One and two year maintenance of treatment effects in the family. *Child & Family Behavior Therapy, 23*(4), 1–20.

Fabiano, G. A., Pelham, W. E., Manos, M. J., Gnagy, E. M., Chronis, A. M., Onyango, AN., … Meichenbaum, D. L. (2004). An evaluation of three time-out procedures for children with attention-deficit/hyperactivity disorder. *Behavior Therapy, 35*(3), 449–469.

Flynn, S. J., Cooper, L. A., & Gary-Webb, T. L. (2013). The role of culture in promoting effective clinical communication, behavior change, and treatment adherence. *The oxford handbook of health communication, behavior change, and treatment adherence* (p. 267).

Gable, R. A., Hester, P. H., Rock, M. L., & Hughes, K. G. (2009). Back to basics rules, praise, ignoring, and reprimands revisited. *Intervention in School and Clinic, 44*(4), 195–205.

Galland, B. C., Taylor, B. J., Elder, D. E., & Herbison, P. (2012). Normal sleep patterns in infants and children: A systematic review of observational studies. *Sleep Medicine Reviews, 16*(3), 213–222.

García Coll, C., Lamberty, G., Jenkins, R., McAdoo, H. P., Crnic, K., Wasik, B. H., & Vazquez García, H. (1996). An integrative model for the study of developmental competencies in minority children. *Child Dev, 67*(5), 1891–1914.

Gershoff, E. T. (2002). Corporal punishment by parents and associated child behaviors and experiences: A meta-analytic and theoretical review. *Psychological Bulletin, 128*(4), 539.

Gibson, M. V., Diaz, V. A., Mainous, A. G., 3rd, & Geesey, M. E. (2005). Prevalence of breastfeeding and acculturation in Hispanics: Results from NHANES 1999-2000 study. *Birth, 32*(2), 93–98. doi:10.1111/j.0730-7659.2005.00351.x.

Ginsburg, K. R. (2007). The importance of play in promoting healthy child development and maintaining strong parent-child bonds. *Pediatrics, 119*(1), 182–191.

Hall, E. (1976). *Beyond culture* (Vol. 222, p. 13). New York: Anchor Books.

Hendy, H. M., & Williams, K. E. (2012). Mother's feeding practices for children 3–10 years of age and their associations with child demographics. *Appetite, 58*(2), 710–716.

Huh, S. Y., Rifas-Shiman, S. L., Taveras, E. M., Oken, E., & Gillman, M. W. (2011). Timing of solid food introduction and risk of obesity in preschool-aged children. *Pediatrics, 127*(3), e544–e551. doi:10.1542/peds.2010-0740.

Horn, I. B., Cheng, T. L., & Joseph, J. (2004). Discipline in the African American Community: The impact of socioeconomic status on beliefs and practices. *Pediatrics, 113*(5), 1–5.

Jenni, O. G., & O'Connor, B. B. (2005). Children's sleep: An interplay between culture and biology. *Pediatrics, 115*(Supp. 1), 204–216.

Johnson, L., Radesky, J., & Zuckerman, B. (2013). Cross-cultural parenting: Reflections on autonomy and interdependence. *Pediatrics, 131*(4), 631–633.

Kazdin, A. E., & Benjet, C. (2003). Spanking children evidence and issues. *Current Directions in Psychological Science, 12*(3), 99–103.

Khandpur, N., Blaine, R. E., Fisher, J. O., & Davison, K. K. (2014). Fathers' child feeding practices: A review of the evidence. *Appetite, 78*, 110–121.

Kim, E., & Hong, S. (2007). First-generation Korean-American parents' perceptions of discipline. *Journal of Professional Nursing, 23*(1), 60–68.

Kuo, A. A., Inkelas, M., Slusser, W. M., Maidenberg, M., & Halfon, N. (2011). Introduction of solid food to young infants. *Maternal and Child Health Journal, 15*(8), 1185–1194. doi:10.1007/s10995-010-0669-5.

Latz, S., Wolf, A. W., & Lozoff, B. (1999). Cosleeping in context: Sleep practices and problems in young children in Japan and the United States. *Archives of Pediatrics & Adolescent Medicine, 153*(4), 339–346.

Lee, A. (2013). *Understanding infant feeding practices among Chinese Mothers in New York city* (Theses paper 2). Syracuse University, Syracuse, NY.

Lee, A., & Brann, L. (2014). Influence of cultural beliefs on infant feeding, postpartum and childcare practices among Chinese-American Mothers in New York city. *Journal of Community Health*, 1–8.

Li, R., Darling, N., Maurice, E., Barker, L., & Grummer-Strawn, L. M. (2005). Breastfeeding rates in the United States by characteristics of the child, mother, or family: The 2002 National Immunization Survey. *Pediatrics, 115*(1), e31–e37.

Lind, J. P., Perrine, C. G., Li, R., Scanlon, K. S., & Grummer-Strawn, L. M. (2014). Racial disparities in access to maternity care practices that support breastfeeding—United States, 2011. *MMWR. Morbidity and Mortality Weekly Report, 63*(33), 725–728.

Liu, X., Liu, L., Owens, J. A., & Kaplan, D. L. (2005). Sleep patterns and sleep problems among schoolchildren in the United States and China. *Pediatrics, 115*(Supp. 1), 241–249.

MacKenzie, M. J., Nicklas, E., Brooks-Gunn, J., & Waldfogel, J. (2015). Spanking and children's externalizing behavior across the first decade of life: Evidence for transactional processes. *Journal of Youth and Adolescence, 44*(3), 658–669.

Mao, A., Burnham, M. M., Goodlin-Jones, B. L., Gaylor, E. E., & Anders, T. F. (2004). A comparison of the sleep–wake patterns of cosleeping and solitary-sleeping infants. *Child Psychiatry and Human Development, 35*(2), 95–105.

Marti, M., Snow, R., Wu, W., & Duch, H. (2015). *The impact of play-based, parent-child intervention on the parent-child interaction of Latino families*. Philadelphia, PA: Society for Research in Child Development.

Matos, M., Torres, R., Santiago, R., Jurado, M., & Rodriguez, I. (2006). Adaptation of parent–child interaction therapy for Puerto Rican families: A preliminary study. *Family Process, 45*(2), 205–222.

McCabe, K., Yeh, M., Garland, A. F., Lau, A. S., & Chavez, G. (2005). The GANA program: A tailoring approach to adapting parent child interaction therapy for Mexican Americans. *Education and Treatment of Children, 28*(2), 111–129.

McCabe, K., Yeh, M., Lau, A. S., & Argote, C. B. (2012). Parent-child interaction therapy for Mexican Americans: Results of a pilot randomized clinical trial at follow-up. *Behavior Therapy, 43*(3), 606–618.

McLoyd, V. C., & Smith, J. (2002). Physical discipline and behavior problems in African American, European American, and Hispanic children: Emotional support as a moderator. *Journal of Marriage and Family, 64*(1), 40–53.

Medoff, D., & Schaefer, C. E. (1993). Children sharing the parental bed: A review of the advantages and disadvantages of cosleeping. *Psychology: A Journal of Human Behavior, 30*(1), 1–9.

Milan, S., Snow, S., & Belay, S. (2007). The context of preschool children's sleep: Racial/ethnic differences in sleep locations, routines, and concerns. *Journal of Family Psychology, 21*(1), 20.

Miller, S. A. (1988). Parents' beliefs about children's cognitive development. *Child Development, 59*(2), 259–285.

Mindell, J. A., Sadeh, A., Kohyama, J., & How, T. H. (2010). Parental behaviors and sleep outcomes in infants and toddlers: A cross-cultural comparison. *Sleep Medicine, 11*(4), 393–399.

Mindell, J. A., Sadeh, A., Kwon, R., & Goh, D. Y. T. (2013). Cross-cultural differences in the sleep of preschool children. *Sleep Medicine, 14*(12), 1283–1289.

Mindell, J. A., Sadeh, A., Wiegand, B., How, T. H., & Goh, D. Y. T. (2010). Cross-cultural differences in infant and toddler sleep. *Sleep Medicine, 11*(3), 274–280.

Morelli, G. A., Rogoff, B., Oppenheim, D., & Goldsmith, D. (1992). Cultural variation in infants' sleeping arrangements: Questions of independence. *Developmental Psychology, 28*(4), 604.

Nielsen, S. J., Rossen, L. M., Harris, D. M., & Ogden, C. L. (2014). Fruit and vegetable consumption of U.S. Youth, 2009–2010. *NCHS Data Brief, 156*, 1–8.

O'Brien, L. M., & Gozal, D. (2004). Neurocognitive dysfunction and sleep in children: From human to rodent. *Pediatric Clinics of North America, 51*(1), 187–202.

Ogden, C. L., Carroll, M. D., Kit, B. K., & Flegal, K. M. (2014). Prevalence of childhood and adult obesity in the United States, 2011–2012. *JAMA, 311*(8), 806–814.

Pai, H., & Contento, I. (2014). Parental perceptions, feeding practices, feeding styles, and level of acculturation of Chinese Americans in relation to their school-age child's weight status. *Appetite, 80*, 174–182.

Palmstierna, P., Sepa, A., & Ludvigsson, J. (2008). Parent perceptions of child sleep: A study of 10 000 Swedish children. *Acta Paediatrica, 97*(12), 1631–1639.

Patterson, G. R. (1979). A performance theory for coercive family interaction. In R. B. Cairns (Ed.), *The analysis of social interactions: Methods, issues, and illustrations* (pp. 119–162). Hillsdale, NJ: Erlbaum.

Perrin, E. M., Rothman, R. L., Sanders, L. M., Skinner, A. C., Eden, S. K., Shintani, A.,…Yin, H. S. (2014). Racial and ethnic differences associated with feeding- and activity-related behaviors in infants. *Pediatrics, 133*(4), e857–e867. doi:10.1542/peds.2013-1326.

Powers, S. W., Chamberlin, L. A., Schaick, K. B., Sherman, S. N., & Whitaker, R. C. (2006). Maternal feeding strategies, child eating behaviors, and child BMI in low-income African-American preschoolers. *Obesity, 14*(11), 2026–2033.

Reeves, E. A., & Woods-Giscombé, C. L. (2014). Infant-feeding practices among African American women: Socio-ecological analysis and implications for practice. *Journal of Transcultural Nursing, 26*(3), 219–226. doi:10.1177/1043659614526244.

Reid, M. J., Webster-Stratton, C., & Beauchaine, T. P. (2001). Parent training in Head Start: A comparison of program response among African American, Asian American, Caucasian, and Hispanic mothers. *Prevention Science, 2*(4), 209–227.

Ren, L., & Pope Edwards, C. (2015). Pathways of influence: Chinese parents' expectations, parenting styles, and child social competence. *Early Child Development and Care, 185*(4), 614–630.

Sadeh, A., Flint-Ofir, E., Tirosh, T., & Tikotzky, L. (2007). Infant sleep and parental sleep-related cognitions. *Journal of Family Psychology, 21*(1), 74.

Sadeh, A., Mindell, J. A., Luedtke, K., & Wiegand, B. (2009). Sleep and sleep ecology in the first 3 years: A web-based study. *Journal of Sleep Research, 18*(1), 60–73.

Sadeh, A., Tikotzky, L., & Scher, A. (2010). Parenting and infant sleep. *Sleep Medicine Reviews, 14*(2), 89–96.

Scheuermann, B. K., & Hall, J. A. (2008). *Positive behavioral supports for the classroom*. Upper Saddle River, NJ: Pearson Higher Ed.

Schuhmann, E. M., Foote, R. C., Eyberg, S. M., Boggs, S. R., & Algina, J. (1998). Efficacy of parent-child interaction therapy: Interim report of a randomized trial with short-term maintenance. *Journal of Clinical Child Psychology, 27*(1), 34–45.

Seid, M., Stevens, G. D., & Varni, J. W. (2003). Parents' perceptions of pediatric primary care quality: Effects of race/ethnicity, language, and access. *Health Services Research, 38*(4), 1009–1032.

Sherry, B., McDivitt, J., Birch, L., Cook, F., Sanders, S., Prish, J. L.,…Scanlon, K. S. (2004). Attitudes, practices, and concerns about child feeding and child weight status among socioeconomically diverse white, Hispanic, and African-American mothers. *Journal of the American Dietetic Association, 104*(2), 215–221.

Suizzo, M. (2007). Parents' goals and values for children dimensions of independence and interdependence across four US ethnic groups. *Journal of Cross-Cultural Psychology, 38*(4), 506–530.

Taveras, E. M., Gillman, M. W., Kleinman, K., Rich-Edwards, J. W., & Rifas-Shiman, S. L. (2010). Racial/ethnic differences in early-life risk factors for childhood obesity. *Pediatrics, 125*(4), 686–695. doi:10.1542/peds.2009-2100.

The Annie E. Casey Foundation. (2014). *The 2014 KIDS COUNT data book*. Baltimore, MA: The Annie E. Casey Foundation.

Tikotzky, L., & Sadeh, A. (2009). Maternal sleep-related cognitions and infant sleep: A longitudinal study from pregnancy through the 1st Year. *Child Development, 80*(3), 860–874.

Tsai, K. M., Telzer, E. H., Gonzales, N. A., & Fuligni, A. J. (2015). Parental cultural socialization of Mexican-American adolescents' family obligation values and behaviors. *Child Development*.

Webster-Stratton, C., Rinaldi, J., & Reid, J. (2011). Long-term outcomes of Incredible Years Parenting Program: Predictors of adolescent adjustment. *Child and Adolescent Mental Health, 16*(1), 38–46.

Wolf, A. W., & Lozoff, B. (1989). Object attachment, thumbsucking, and the passage to sleep. *Journal of the American Academy of Child and Adolescent Psychiatry, 28*(2), 287–292.

Wolf, T. L., McLaughlin, T. F., & Williams, R. L. (2006). Time-out interventions and strategies: A brief review and recommendations. *International Journal of Special Education, 21*(3), 22–29.

Wu, P., Robinson, C. C., Yang, C., Hart, C. H., Olsen, S. F., Porter, CL.,…Wu, X. (2002). Similarities and differences in mothers' parenting of preschoolers in China and the United States. *International Journal of Behavioral Development, 26*(6), 481–491.

Chapter 9
Funding, Financing, and Investing in Integrated Early Childhood Mental Health Services in Primary Care Settings

Ayelet Talmi, Melissa Buchholz, and Emily F. Muther

Abstract Integrating early childhood mental health services into primary care settings holds promise for increasing access to high quality healthcare services. Such services have the potential to prevent the development of later difficulties, promote health and well-being, identify early difficulties and address them when they first emerge, and treat disruptions and disorders in early childhood, including family-level factors that impact development. Establishing sustainable integrated early childhood behavioral health services requires leveraging resources and braiding and blending funding streams to create a comprehensive model of care that will meet the needs of young children and their families. Long-term sustainability depends upon advancing the "Four Ps": *procedures*, *practice*, *payment*, and *policy*. This chapter details *procedures* for service delivery and billing that comply with healthcare regulations and allow continued growth and program innovation and characterizes the unique elements within the *practice* of integrated early childhood mental health services including a focus on prevention, health promotion, and universal access to high-quality care. In the current landscape of rapid healthcare reform and transformation, *payment* and compensation for services rendered and future innovations in service delivery are integrally linked to *policy* changes that are designed to secure integrated early childhood services. Beyond fee-for-service options, truly sustainable integrated early childhood behavioral health will likely rely on bundled payment models where early childhood mental health services are packaged within high-quality primary care for children, and capitated/per member per month (PMPM) rates reflect investments in prevention, health promotion, psychosocial screening processes, and interventions.

A. Talmi, Ph.D. (✉) • M. Buchholz, Psy.D. • E.F. Muther, Ph.D.
University of Colorado School of Medicine, Children's Hospital Colorado,
Aurora, CO, USA
e-mail: ayelet.talmi@ucdenver.edu; melissa.buchholz@ucdenver.edu;
emily.muther@childrenscolorado.org

© Springer International Publishing Switzerland 2016
R.D. Briggs (ed.), *Integrated Early Childhood Behavioral Health in Primary Care*, DOI 10.1007/978-3-319-31815-8_9

Keywords Early childhood • Behavioral health integration • Integrated care • Sustainability • Pediatric primary care • Healthcare financing • Payment reform • Prevention • Health promotion

Introduction

"This all sounds great," you say, "but how in the world are we going to pay for it?" In this chapter, we discuss the challenges and opportunities in funding and sustaining early childhood integrated behavioral health programs and services. We begin by detailing the current healthcare funding landscape and subsequently describe integrated early childhood behavioral health services and the funding mechanisms used to deliver them. After providing an example of efforts to develop and sustain an integrated behavioral health services program, we conclude with general recommendations and strategies for developing and sustaining integrated early childhood services.

Establishing sustainable integrated early childhood behavioral health services in primary care settings requires leveraging resources and braiding and blending funding streams to create a comprehensive model of care that will meet the needs of young children and their families. We suggest that long-term sustainability depends upon advancing the "Four Ps": *procedures*, *practice*, *payment*, and *policy*. As will be detailed below, *procedures* for service delivery and billing must be clearly delineated, implemented, tracked, and adjusted in order to create funding streams that comply with healthcare regulations and allow continued growth and program innovation. The *practice* of integrated early childhood mental health services is unique, with a focus on prevention, health promotion, and universal access to high-quality care. Securing additional funds through grants and contracts may be necessary during early stages of program design and implementation, or during phases when new services are added to ensure *payment* and compensation, both for services rendered and future efforts. The fourth "p," *policy*, is essential to the long-term sustainability of integrated early childhood services.

The Healthcare Landscape

The Patient Protection and Affordable Care Act (ACA; Patient Protection and Affordable Care Act, 2010) includes mental health services among the essential health benefits provided through the expansion of Medicaid and the health insurance exchanges established at the state level. Despite the inclusion of mental and behavioral health services in the core package of health benefits, state plans and insurance exchanges vary widely regarding which services are funded and to what extent. Consequently, funding integrated mental health services presents numerous

challenges. Foremost among these are the significant billing and regulatory requirements for reimbursement of mental and behavioral health services provided in the
context of primary care, including limitations on same day billing for physical and
mental health services, mental health carve-outs, non-reimbursable case management activities, and lack of incentives for screening, health promotion, and prevention efforts (American Academy of Child and Adolescent Psychiatry Committee on
Health Care Access and Economics, 2009; Mauch, Kautz, & Smith, 2008).

Establishing and sustaining funding for integrated early childhood mental health
services is an even more complex proposition. Integrated early childhood mental
health services are, by design, intended to promote health and well-being through
prevention, early identification, and initiation of treatment before serious disruptions
and disorders emerge. In contrast to this focus on prevention, the vast majority of
healthcare services are diagnosis and disorder driven within a system that is designed
to identify and treat problems that already exist and qualify for a given diagnosis.
Providing early childhood integrated behavioral health services, which are inher-
ently prevention focused, has the potential to alter developmental trajectories so that
young children never reach diagnostic thresholds. As such, the vast majority of these
services are not eligible for reimbursement within the current system.

Procedures: Funding for Services Delivered in Primary Care Settings

In this section we provide an overview of billing strategies and funding mechanisms
for service delivery within primary care settings including fee-for-service (FFS),
Current Procedural Terminology (CPT®) Codes, Health & Behavior (H&B) Codes,
mental health carve-outs, and bundled payments. Understanding the intricacies of
billing and reimbursement *procedures* is necessary for designing, implementing,
and funding integrated early childhood behavioral health services.

Fee-for-Service

One of the most common ways of paying for healthcare services today is the FFS
system, where services are unbundled and healthcare providers bill and are paid
for each discrete component, procedures, or service separately (Miller, 2009). For
example, physical exams, immunizations, lab tests, and other procedures are
billed individually depending on what is delivered during a healthcare visit.
Currently, fee-for-service is the most common financial payment model for individuals with behavioral health needs (Barlow, Wright, Sheasby, Turner, &
Hainsworth, 2002). This model can be problematic for services provided within
primary care because many states have policies prohibiting billing for a primary

care visit and a behavioral health visit in the same clinic on the same day ("same day billing"), impeding interdisciplinary and coordinated care, the very cornerstone of integrated care (American Association of Community Psychiatrists, 2002; Monson, Sheldon, Ivey, Kinman, & Beacham, 2012). Furthermore, these practices are limited because of separate public and private payers and inconsistent rules regarding who is able to bill for what service. This artificial separation of physical and behavioral healthcare, mainly through mental health carve-outs, prevents primary care providers from billing for mental health screening and intervention (Barlow et al., 2002).

In the case of integrated early childhood mental health services, the FFS model with a carve-out for mental and behavioral healthcare is especially problematic. As previously mentioned, young children and their caregivers may experience symptoms that manifest as functional impairments without reaching diagnostic thresholds that make them eligible for services through FFS payment models, dependent on diagnosis.

Health and Behavior Codes

In 2002, the health and behavior (H&B) assessment and intervention codes were approved for inclusion into the current CPT® system (Drotar, 2012). The CPT® codes were developed in 1966 by the American Medical Association (AMA) to define and document medical procedures and services (Lines, Tynan, Angalet, & Pendley, 2012; Mauch et al., 2008). These codes are utilized for documentation and as the primary method by which third-party reimbursement for services is obtained in a FFS landscape. Psychologists have historically used mental health CPT® codes to bill for the therapy and assessment services they provide. However, while these codes can be relevant to the practice of psychologists in pediatric primary care, they are not sufficient for documenting the entirety of the work performed by these clinicians (Lines et al., 2012). Furthermore, the early childhood services provided by psychologists in pediatric primary care are often not associated with psychopathology or mental health diagnoses of either the patient or the family. Consequently, traditional methods of billing that focus on identification of mental health diagnoses do not encompass the broad scope of early childhood work conducted in pediatric primary care, and the H&B codes address many of these concerns.

The H&B codes are a set of codes intended for the use by nonphysician providers who provide assessment and treatment for biopsychosocial factors related to a patient's physical health diagnosis (American Psychological Association, 2004). A significant distinction for the use of H&B codes is that behavioral health providers using the codes are associating a medical diagnosis to their billing, rather than a mental health diagnosis (see Table 9.1). Thus, preventive mental health efforts, as long as they are associated with a medical diagnosis, may be covered. The reimbursement for the services billed with H&B codes is paid under the medical benefits of a patient's insurance and not the mental health benefits. Mental health carve-outs will be addressed in more detail below.

Table 9.1 Selected Current Procedural Terminology (CPT®) and billing codes used in early childhood integrated behavioral healthcare

CPT® or procedure code	Definition[a]	Service description	Billing details
96110	Developmental screening (e.g., developmental milestone survey, speech and language delay screen), with scoring and documentation, per standardized instrument	Developmental screening (including screening for autism, developmental domains, language delays, etc.) at well-child visits using a standardized instrument	1 unit = 1 screening; approximately $9.65/screening event; limits on frequency of screenings vary by state
96111	Developmental testing, (includes assessment of motor, language, social, adaptive, and/or cognitive functioning by standardized developmental instruments) with interpretation and report	Expanded assessment/testing of development at well-child or follow-up visits using standardized instruments	1 unit = 1 assessment event; approximately $122/assessment event
96127 (new code in 2015)	Brief emotional/behavioral assessment (e.g., depression inventory, attention-deficit/hyperactivity disorder [ADHD] scale), with scoring and documentation, per standardized instrument	Brief assessment of emotional/behavioral issues using a screening instrument (e.g., for depression, attention deficit/ hyperactivity, anxiety)	1 unit = 1 screening; approximately $5.00/screening instrument; limits on frequency of screenings vary by state
96150	Health and behavior assessment (e.g., health-focused clinical interview, behavioral observations, psychophysiological monitoring, health-oriented questionnaires), face-to-face with the patient; initial assessment	Assessment of health concerns; medical diagnoses; fussiness; feeding difficulties; lactation issues; growth/physical development issues; congenital anomaly, etc.	1 unit = 15 min; approximately $21/ unit
96151	Health and behavior assessment (e.g., health-focused clinical interview, behavioral observations, psychophysiological monitoring, health-oriented questionnaires), face-to-face with the patient; re-assessment	Re-assessment of health and medical concerns after a period of intervention and/or a period of time since initial assessment	1 unit = 15 min; approximately $20/ unit
96152	Health and behavior intervention, face-to-face; individual	Intervention around health and medical concerns; typically not used in early childhood because young children are not seen without caregivers though if direct care only to patient, use this code	1 unit = 15 min; approximately $19/ unit

(continued)

Table 9.1 (continued)

CPT® or procedure code	Definition[a]	Service description	Billing details
96154	Health and behavior intervention, face-to-face; family (with the patient present)	Intervention around health and medical concerns with the family and patient present at well-child, sick, or follow-up visits	1 unit = 15 min; approximately $19/unit
H0002	Behavioral health screening to determine eligibility for admission to treatment program	Initial screening to establish eligibility for services (e.g., recruiting for Healthy Steps)	1 unit = 1 encounter; reimbursement unknown
H0023	Behavioral health outreach service (planned approach to reach a targeted population)	Outreach to a population to engage in behavioral health services; used to inform and engage in available services	1 unit = 1 encounter; reimbursement unknown
H0025	Behavioral health prevention education service (delivery of services with target population to affect knowledge, attitude, and/or behavior)	Psychoeducation; developmental support; assessment and intervention around environmental and familial factors including caregiver mental health issues at well-child, sick and follow-up visits	1 unit = 1 encounter; reimbursement unknown
G8431 (positive) G8510 (negative)	Procedural code for medical provider/setting screening for maternal mood and anxiety concerns using a standardized instrument with documentation of results (positive/negative) and intervention offered	Screening for pregnancy-related mood and anxiety at well-child visits between birth and 4 months	1 unit = 1 screening instrument; approximately $10/screening; frequency, eligible settings, and reimbursement amounts vary by state

[a]Current Procedural Terminology (CPT®) copyright, 2014. American Medical Association. All rights reserved

Note: CPT® code relative value calculator is available at: https://ocm.ama-assn.org/OCM/CPTRelativeValueSearch.do?submitbutton=accept

While the approval of the health and behavior codes was an important develop-ment for integrated behavioral health in medical settings, numerous barriers to bill-ing and reimbursement significantly limit their utility (Talmi & Fazio, 2012). As a physical health diagnosis is required for the use of H&B codes, these still do not adequately address the true preventive nature of early childhood behavioral health programs. When a child does have a physical health diagnosis, and a provider can use H&B codes, there are still challenges, including inadequate and inconsistent reimbursement practices that vary by state and type of insurer. As an example, Colorado's Medicaid Program does not recognize psychologists and other licensed mental health professionals as authorized provider types when they bill using health and behavior codes, which means that these "non-authorized provider types" cannot be reimbursed for services rendered (Talmi & Fazio, 2012).

Mental and Behavioral Health Carve-Outs

Beyond the challenges posed by FFS, CPT codes, and H&B codes, the administra-tion of physical and behavioral health is often based in multiple state agencies, which complicates policy action on issues ranging from the elimination of "carve-outs" to the promotion of innovative payment systems (Ader et al., 2015). Data from 2011 indicated that 24 US state Medicaid programs carved out at least a portion of their behavioral health benefits (Kaiser Commission on Medicaid and the Uninsured, 2011; Swartz & Morrissey, 2012). Mental health carve-outs delineate mental and behavioral health services that are provided and paid for in a system separate from physical health services. Within this model, mental and behavioral services, provid-ers, and settings are managed and administered separately, typically requiring pre-authorizations for care, paneling or credentialing of providers with mental health licenses, and benefits that cannot be accessed or provided in physical health set-tings. Practitioners with mental health specialty credentials are favored in carve-out networks, which often exclude primary care providers (Mauch, 2002). The presence of behavioral health carve-outs has impeded the delivery of integrated behavioral healthcare as primary care providers are often unable to obtain reimbursement for treatment related to mental health diagnoses (Kathol, Butler, McAlpine, & Kane, 2010; Kathol, Degruy, & Rollman, 2014). A number of sources have demonstrated how carve-outs have the significant potential to result in more fragmented and uncoordinated healthcare (Ader et al., 2015; American Psychiatric Association, 2002; Kathol et al., 2010; Summer & Hoadley, 2014). Primary care providers who are unable to get reimbursed because they are not in the carve-out network may not have incentive to evaluate the need for behavioral health intervention for their patients. This reimbursement barrier impacts the primary care provider's ability to focus on prevention and early intervention, and as a result, conditions are identified at a much later point, where the opportunity to have the greatest impact is decreased (Ader et al., 2015). Additionally, carving out behavioral health services may involve developing separate contracts with external companies who are contracted to meet the behavioral health needs of a segment of the population receiving physical health services. These subcontracts create an artificial separation between physical and mental health services making it challenging for health systems, and the providers that work within them, to manage population health outcomes when they are not necessarily responsible for 100 % of the benefits and coverage for their members.

Other Models of Care and Payment: Beyond the Fee-for-Service and CPT Landscape

It is well known that healthcare costs have grown at an unsustainable rate. Efforts to reduce cost by improving coordination and efficiency of care are exemplified in the emergence of accountable care organizations (ACOs), patient-centered medical homes (PCMHs), and other global or bundled payment arrangements with incentives that reward high value healthcare (Selker, Kravitz, & Gallagher, 2014) and depart from the traditional FFS model dependent on diagnosis. The rollout of healthcare reform legislation includes new approaches to care and payment models with a focus on value-based versus volume-based care and payment (Chesney & Lindeke, 2012). One successful approach to ensuring sustainable early childhood services in pediatric primary care is to use capitated funding mechanisms to negotiate contracts with behavioral health entities to embed qualified and experienced behavioral health clinicians into primary care (Cohen, Davis, Hall, Gilchrist, & Miller, 2015). Behavioral health managed care entities with capitated contracts have an interest in increasing their penetration rates to serve the targeted number of individuals in their catchment areas. Behavioral health clinicians working in pediatric primary care have an opportunity to reach a large number of children and families who can be counted as receiving services under capitated behavioral health plans (Talmi & Fazio, 2012). Many states have behavioral health organizations (BHOs) that fund clinicians to deliver mental health services in primary care settings. By co-locating a full-time behavioral health clinician into primary care, the mental health center can better serve its target population within a designated geographic region, increase penetration rates, and, thereby, fulfill contractual requirements with Medicaid (Talmi & Fazio, 2012).

ACOs are provider-based organizations that were created to improve care coordination and reduce redundancy and waste by assuming responsibility and accountability for the quality, cost, and comprehensive care of a defined population of patients (American Academy of Pediatrics, 2011; Chesney & Lindeke, 2012; National Committee for Quality Assurance, 2010). Within the legislation of the ACA is language calling for the Department of Health & Human Services to establish a Pediatric Demonstration Project to promote ACOs in Medicaid and Children's Health Insurance Programs (CHIPs) between 2012 and 2016 (American Academy of Pediatrics, 2011; Chesney & Lindeke, 2012). Unlike the current FFS reimbursement model of healthcare, the ACO payment structure is based on payment for quality of care, instead of rewarding high volume and quantity of care. ACOs apply the responsibility for costs and quality across a defined population to a network of providers who offer health *and* behavioral health services, with an increased emphasis on prevention and population health (Fisher & Shortell, 2010). Financial incentives are directed toward care teams who keep their patients healthy by providing safe, effective, and efficient care (Chesney & Lindeke, 2012; Miller, 2009). A pediatric ACO in Ohio, serving a primarily Medicaid population, was found to reduce the growth costs compared with FFS Medicaid and averaged less cost than managed care Medicaid during a 5-year period (Kelleher et al., 2015). This model also improved the quality of care for children and families covered by Medicaid (Kelleher et al., 2015). However, it is important to recognize that the vast majority of ACOs focus on older adults, where it is far easier to obtain short-term cost savings and improvements in health via the provision of coordinated care. Furthermore, most ACOs today continue to segment out the provision of mental healthcare, missing an opportunity for true integration (Lewis et al., 2014).

Per Member Per Month (PMPM) structures, common in recent alternative payment models including ACOs, address some of the challenges related to FFS payments. This model is an alternative payment form in which a practice or provider is given a set amount of money each month to provide an agreed upon range of services for the patients enrolled in this program for the period of time covered by the agreement (Rosenthal, 2008). Therefore, PMPM incentivizes providers to implement wellness strategies that keep their patients healthier and reduce the need for expensive acute care services. Consequently, capitation models of payment are designed to control the number of episodes of care as well as the cost of individual episodes (Miller, 2009). The idea behind capitated payment is for a practice to receive a single payment to cover all services their patients need during a specific period of time, regardless of how many or few episodes of care the patients receive (Miller, 2009). However, traditional capitation models may disincentivize providers from enrolling patients who require expensive care because the amount of payment they receive is the same regardless of how sick or well the patients are (Miller, 2009).

While the value of behavioral health in primary care for children and families is well established, the challenges of justifying its unreimbursed costs remain an issue. Further exploration of models that allow for bundled payments for specific early childhood behavioral health and primary care services is needed. This would allow for reimbursement for team-based care, and incentives for improved health outcomes (Monson et al., 2012).

Practice: Integrated Early Childhood Behavioral Health Services

In the next section, we provide examples of early childhood integrated behavioral health *practices* and describe the funding mechanisms and financing strategies used in primary care settings to deliver and pay for these services, which include screening, care coordination, and intervention. Universal screening efforts provide information about young child and caregiver well-being and facilitate early identification and intervention when concerns arise. Care coordination is central to high quality primary care services and promotes connection to resources, communication among professionals, tracking of referral uptake, and successful management of health and environmental factors that impact well-being. Lastly, the Healthy Steps for Young Children Program, Breastfeeding Management Clinic, and other early childhood behavioral health interventions around challenging behaviors and identified difficulties represent the continuum of integrated interventions from prevention and health promotion to targeted, problem-based consultations. See Table 9.2 for examples of early childhood integrated practices and billing elements.

Screening Processes

Developmental screening Universal screening is an important component of integrated early childhood mental health services in primary care settings. Screening facilitates early identification, early referral, and early intervention for a variety of conditions, which if left unaddressed, may lead to more significant disruptions later in a child or family's life. The American Academy of Pediatrics recommends the use of a standardized screening tool for development as part of well-child care (Pediatrics, 2006). Routine developmental screening can be reimbursed when billed under the CPT® code of 96110. Reimbursement rates vary by state and by insurance type, with a national average of $10/screening encounter (see Table 9.1).

Within an early childhood integrated behavioral health services program, universal developmental screening helps ensure that those children requiring referrals for evaluation and intervention receive timely access to care. Ideally, universal screening processes are built into the primary care clinic's workflow, including training for providers on the use of various screening instruments, distribution of screening instruments to families for completion, scoring, feedback of screening results, and documentation of screening efforts and collateral services. Unfortunately, while rates of universal screening continue to increase, the majority of pediatric primary care providers report that they do not use standardized developmental screening (Radecki, Sand-Loud, O'Connor, Sharp, & Olson, 2011), relying instead on surveillance methods. Even when screening instruments are used, many children with abnormal screening results do not get referred for a more comprehensive evaluation (Halfon, Stevens, Larson, & Olson, 2011; King et al. 2010) until their delays manifest more profoundly or when they experience significant disruptions in functional abilities (Rosenberg, Zhang, & Robinson, 2008).

Integrated early childhood mental health services offer a possible solution to screening challenges. When screening results fall in the abnormal range, primary care providers may utilize the services of an early childhood mental health consultant to assist in discussing the identified concern with the family, making appropriate referrals, ensuring connection with necessary services and systems, and providing follow-up support to the family (Briggs et al., 2012).

Increasing the incidence of screening rates in primary care settings is strengthened by collaborative efforts with practices and statewide early childhood partners.

Table 9.2 Coding and billing case examples

Demographics	Presenting concern	Intervention	Visit type	Diagnosis	CPT code billed
18 month old	Child score on a developmental screening indicates risk for speech delay	Reviewed results of screening with family; Discussed family's concerns about development; Facilitated a referral for an early intervention evaluation	Well-child visit	Routine well-child visit (V20.2)	96110
15 day old Born at 36 weeks gestation	Mother struggling with breastfeeding; Infant is very sleepy at the breast; Mother is highly anxious about being able to successfully breastfeed	Screened for pregnancy-related depression; Reviewed connection between maternal mental health and self-care with successful breastfeeding; Discussed strategies to manage anxiety; Provided mental health referrals for mother	Lactation consultation	Feeding difficulty in a newborn (P92.9)	96150
3 month old	Weight gain continues to be slow; Mother is depressed and anxious	Facilitated referral to mental health provider in mother's community; Reviewed importance of self-care strategies for mother	Lactation consultation	Slow weight gain in a newborn (P92.6)	96154
9 month old	Healthy baby; Parents have a lot of questions about what to expect	Enrolled in Healthy Steps; Provided family with anticipatory guidance about topics such as child proofing, language development, gross motor development	Well-child visit	Routine well-child visit (V20.2)	H0025

(continued)

Table 9.2 (continued)

Demographics	Presenting concern	Intervention	Visit type	Diagnosis	CPT code billed
4 month old	Elevated maternal depression screening score	Evaluated maternal mental health, social support resources, and need for further mental health support; Facilitated referral to mental health resources; Plan to follow-up with family at 6-month well-child visit	Well-child visit	Routine well-child visit (V20.2)	H0025 G8431 (Medical Provider code for screening)
2 month old	Fussy baby	Medical explanations for fussiness ruled out by medical provider; Provide psychoeducation about infant crying; Support caregiver and strategize about ways to address fussiness	Same day sick visit	Fussiness in a baby (R68.12)	96150
18 month old	Healthy child Concerns about aggressive behavior	Evaluate onset of behavior and contributing factors; Provide caregiver with strategies for addressing behavior; Schedule follow-up to ensure improvement in behavior	Well-child visit	Routine well-child visit (V20.2)	Not billable

Early childhood mental health clinicians can offer support with implementing screening protocols in the context of the PCMH and can assist the primary care practice in referring families for further evaluation.

Nationally, the Assuring Better Child Health and Development (ABCD) Program was developed to help state systems improve provision of early childhood developmental services (Berry, Krutz, Langner et al., 2008). States that participate in ABCD develop strategies to encourage universal use of standardized developmental tools in primary care settings, including advocating for reimbursement for screening (National Academy for State Health Policy, 2009). Integrated early childhood mental health services related to screening are documented in the child's health record and care is coordinated among systems and service providers to address possible developmental delays (Talmi et al., 2014).

On the Ground Example

Colorado received support from the National ABCD program from 2007 to 2010 and provided training and technical assistance to primary care providers across the state in implementation of developmental screening and referral processes. Colorado ABCD continues to support primary care providers with implementation of screening and referral processes, but does so in collaboration with community early childhood stakeholders in order to ensure that providers are supported in their screening efforts. Recently, Colorado ABCD funded early childhood mental health clinicians in three community pediatric practices to support screening and referral processes. With the assistance of the mental health providers, referrals to local Early Intervention programs increased dramatically (Buchholz, Dunn, & Badwan, 2012).

Screening for pregnancy-related mood and anxiety disorders Pediatric primary care is a uniquely appropriate setting to screen for pregnancy-related depression (Health Team Works, 2014) and other parental mental health issues. The mental health and well-being of caregivers directly impacts child development, particularly during infancy and early childhood when babies are entirely dependent on adults for their care (Murray, Fearon, & Cooper, 2015). Ideally, primary care providers screen for and consider parental mental health as they assess environmental and social determinants of health during well-child visits. Importantly, caregivers are more likely to attend visits at their infant's primary care setting in the weeks and months following birth than to be seen in any other healthcare setting. Therefore, the likelihood of being able to intervene early with caregivers who are struggling with pregnancy-related mood disorders increases when screening occurs in the context of pediatric primary care.

Integrated early childhood mental health consultants play an essential role in screening, identifying, triaging, and treating parental mental health issues that emerge when young children are seen for well-child checks. Screening processes around pregnancy-related mood and anxiety disorders include distribution of screening tools at infant well-child visits from newborn through the 4-month well-child check and beyond, scoring and providing feedback on screening results, and developing protocols for elevated scores that include referrals, care coordination, and access to resources. In some states and with some insurance companies, billing for pregnancy-related mood disorder screening is allowable under screening codes (e.g., CPT® G8431 for a positive screen and CPT® G8510 for a negative screen) across various healthcare settings including primary care, obstetrics, and even in community-based organizations. Typically, approval for reimbursement depends upon negotiations with managed care organizations and state agencies responsible for administering Medicaid benefits.

Integrated early childhood mental health consultants are instrumental in establishing screening processes that support the identification and treatment of parental mental health and environmental issues impacting the well-being of young children and their families. Primary care settings are more likely to be amenable to screening for parental mental health and environmental issues when they can readily refer families with identified difficulties to an early childhood mental health consultant practicing within the primary care setting (Lovell, Roemer, & Talmi, 2014). Reimbursement provides an additional incentive for engaging in screening practices.

On the Ground Example

The DC Collaborative for Mental Health in Pediatric Primary Care ("the Collaborative") aims to improve the integration of mental health in primary pediatric care for children in the District of Columbia. Comprised of professional organizations, health care entities, governmental agencies, and legal partners, and guided by an interdisciplinary advisory group, the Collaborative has been integrally involved in the successful efforts to ensure pediatric primary care providers in the District of Columbia can be reimbursed by Medicaid (FFS and Managed Care Organizations or MCOs) for administering early childhood and perinatal mental health screens at well-child visits. Currently, providers are reimbursed for administering behavioral and/or developmental screens, including the Edinburgh, using 96110, and positive screens are indicated with the modifier "TS." Providers are reimbursed at $10.30 for each screener.

Screening for parental mental health issues in pediatric settings is becoming a more established practice despite the significant barriers to paying for such services. Examples of two generation payment models (Golden & Fortuny, 2011), where services for parents and children are reimbursed regardless of the setting in which these services occur, provide an avenue for integrated early childhood mental health consultants to deliver comprehensive care to young children and their families from within primary care setting.

Care Coordination

Care coordination is a necessary component of high quality primary care settings and medical homes. These settings are charged with coordinating treatment and services across subspecialties and settings in which patients are seen, enhancing communication among families, health professionals, and other providers, triaging care, managing and creating access to vital information, and identifying appropriate resources and ensuring that families successfully access those resources. Care coordination is not typically reimbursed when provided in the context of primary care settings. Recent innovations in financing have incentivized the PCMH with per-member/per-month payments when the practice is able to demonstrate that it performs care coordination functions that meet payment standards. The care coordination efforts of integrated early childhood mental health consultants can be used to demonstrate eligibility for additional per-member/per-month incentives. Integrated early childhood services are frequently blended with other services and resources (e.g., nurse phone lines, social work, family navigation) to create a care coordination approach that directly impacts the quality of care children and families receive.

> **On the Ground Example**
>
> New York's Department of Health is implementing the Children's Health Home Program. Health homes are intended to provide comprehensive and coordinated care in order to meet the complex needs of children and their families. Physical and behavioral health are integrated in these settings and care is child/family-centered. Potential Health Homes must complete an application and meet specific criteria to become designated and receive financial benefits. New York anticipates children will begin to be enrolled in the Health Home program in late 2016.

Integrated Early Childhood Services

Healthy Steps for Young Children The Healthy Steps for Young Children Program (Barth, 2010; Minkovitz et al., 2007) is an integrated program in which infant mental health principles are infused into primary care settings. Healthy Steps is intended to provide families with comprehensive information about development and behavior via an integrated approach to primary healthcare. A Healthy Steps Specialist (an individual with expertise in child development) partners with a primary care provider to collaboratively provide enhanced well-child care to families enrolled in the program (Buchholz & Talmi, 2012). In addition to visits in the primary care clinic, home visits are offered one to two times per year and give the Healthy Steps Specialist a chance to build supportive relationships with families and to strengthen the link between the family and the primary care practice. Healthy Steps also offers parenting groups designed to provide anticipatory guidance, support, and developmental information to families. The Healthy Steps Program has been shown to impact parenting outcomes (e.g., increasing parent confidence, reduced harsh discipline strategies, and increased satisfaction with well-child care) as well as child outcomes (e.g., increased attendance at well-child checks, more timely immunizations; Minkovitz et al., 2007).

The Healthy Steps Program has been able to grow and advance toward sustainability by identifying, accessing, and leveraging federal funds to provide integrated services in the context of primary care. Long-term sustainability of these programs continues to be an important consideration and will need to be addressed in the coming years if the program is to be expanded (Barth, 2010). See Chap. 5 in this volume for more information on Healthy Steps future sustainability plans.

Breastfeeding Management Clinic The breastfeeding experience for the mother and infant is often complicated by a constellation of challenges that are difficult for medical clinicians to treat on their own. Numerous biopsychosocial influences can affect nursing success—infertility, pregnancy course, family circumstances, prematurity, siblings, and mental health issues in the family. In our experience, providing breastfeeding consultation and support in the primary care clinic with an integrated mental health team helps address the complex nature of the early postpartum period. Our "Trifecta Breastfeeding Approach" is an integrated mental health model that meets families' needs by addressing the infant's medical care, functional breastfeeding challenges, and the developing mother–infant relationship, including the screening of concurrent pregnancy-related mood disorders (Bunik, Dunn, Watkins, & Talmi, 2014).

The early childhood psychologist who practices in this clinic bills using H&B codes for assessment (96150) at a family's first visit to clinic and family intervention with patient present (96154) for subsequent visits. The H&B codes can be used in this setting because they are associated with a specific medical diagnosis, most often feeding difficulties or poor weight gain in a newborn. Using this strategy, about half of what is billed by the early childhood psychologist is reimbursed. The reimbursement for these codes comes solely from private insurers because Colorado Medicaid does not currently reimburse H&B codes. Notably, grant funding supported the development and initial implementation of the Trifecta Model, allowing us to formulate sustainability strategies and test billing and reimbursement options. This particular service lends itself to negotiating bundled rates for the highly specialized care provided with the Trifecta Model.

Payment and *Policy*: **Sustainability and Systems-Building**

Despite the numerous barriers to funding and sustainability, integrated mental health programs in pediatric and family medicine settings exist and thrive, amassing evidence regarding their viability and value (Bunik & Talmi, 2012; Cohen et al., 2015; Committee on Child Health Financing, 2013; Mauch et al., 2008; Talmi, Stafford, & Buchholz, 2009). With respect to *payment*, strategies for funding integrated care programs and services range from obtaining philanthropic and state or federal funding to partnering with ACOs and BHOs contracted to provide mental health services. Programs embedded in academic medical centers may access training funds to support professional development for both mental health and primary healthcare providers. Community pediatric settings accepting a wide range of insurance plans may seek reimbursement for services rendered by mental health professionals through "incident to" billing or through direct billing of mental health procedural codes. At the federal level, funding may be available for innovative programs that demonstrate the cost-effectiveness of integrated behavioral health services though obtaining such funding often requires having existing partnerships and collaborations among health system stakeholders. The following is an example of our efforts to build a sustainable integrated behavioral health services program at Children's Hospital Colorado using the strategies described above.

Project CLIMB Project CLIMB (Consultation Liaison In Mental Health and Behavior), an integrated mental health services program located in the Child Health Clinic at Children's Hospital Colorado, utilizes a number of the strategies detailed previously for sustainability. The program was initially funded through generous grants from The Colorado Health Foundation and Rose Community Foundation, large, private Colorado-based foundations interested in improving the health and well-being of Colorado's citizens. Both foundations were interested in creating access to mental health services for underserved Coloradans, improving the health of Coloradans, and training healthcare providers across the State in identification and treatment of mental health issues. An Access Grant through the American Academy of Child and Adolescent Psychiatry enabled us to conduct a small program evaluation with both family and provider surveys. Funding from Liberty Mutual Foundation, the philanthropic arm of Liberty Mutual Insurance, and Denver Post Season to Share, the leading Colorado newspaper's community grant-making campaign, provided additional support for clinical and training services. A one-year grant from Roots and Branches, a program of Rose Community Foundation designed to cultivate philanthropic leadership in young professionals, provided pilot funding to initiate our group programs and services. These programs are now sustained through braided and blended funding including federal MIECHV funding, departmental and institutional support, and donor-directed giving through the Children's Hospital Colorado Foundation. MIECHV funding has enabled us to expand the Healthy Steps for Young Children Program both within our clinic and across Colorado to the highest risk communities statewide.

In partnership with a Behavioral Health Organization (in Colorado, BHOs hold the Medicaid contracts for providing capitated mental health services), we hired a full-time licensed clinician, paid for by the BHO, to work in our primary care setting. This clinician works alongside our faculty and trainees, providing additional services and supports to the families and providers in our setting. The clinician counts contacts in the clinic toward required penetration rates delineated in the BHO contract with Medicaid.

After implementing universal screening processes and tracking revenue generated through screening reimbursements, the Department of Pediatrics at the University of Colorado School of Medicine assumed the cost of two part-time faculty members, a psychologist and a psychiatrist, in order to continue the program's long-standing training efforts. At present, this funding is allocated to fund 10 % each of four psychologists and 30 % total of two psychiatrists. We successfully leveraged faculty time to supervise trainees (postdoctoral fellows, psychology interns, psychology externs, and psychiatry residents) who provide additional services to clinic, increasing access to integrated early childhood mental health services and providing opportunities to cultivate a well-trained workforce.

Policy Efforts to develop, implement, evaluate, and sustain integrated behavioral health services in primary care settings abound. As programs become established and identify successful models for service delivery and sustainability, information about needs, gaps, and effective strategies is accumulated and can be used to shape and inform advocacy agendas and the fourth "p," *policy*. Advocacy and policy efforts create environments in which innovative services and practices can exist, thrive, and ultimately, transform systems of care. Advocacy for integrated early childhood services involves:

1. Identifying funding streams that pay for prevention and health promotion services,
2. Supporting early childhood mental health and behavioral services for the majority of young children and families who do not meet diagnostic criteria for mental or behavioral health conditions, but who would benefit from support, resources, and interventions to help maintain optimal developmental trajectories,
3. Promoting two-generation/multi-generation, family-level services,
4. Advancing healthcare practice and systems transformation that comprehensively integrates and pays for early childhood mental health services in the context of primary care.

On the Ground Example

The DC Collaborative for Mental Health in Pediatric Primary Care also secured funding from the DC Department of Behavioral Health to implement DC Mental Health Access in Pediatrics (DC MAP). DC MAP provides free mental health telephonic consultation services for pediatric primary care providers, and is staffed by a dedicated team of mental health professionals. The team can consult regarding questions ranging from community referrals and resources to medication management, including early childhood mental health inquiries.

Conclusions

Integrating early childhood mental health services into primary care settings holds promise for increasing access to high quality healthcare services that have the potential to prevent the development of later difficulties, promote health and well-being, identify early difficulties and provide services and supports to address them when they first emerge, and treat disruptions and disorders in early childhood, including family-level factors that impact development.

Supporting early childhood behavioral health integration into pediatric primary care requires transformations to healthcare practice and payment systems in both the public and private sectors. These changes include expanding coverage within FFS models for codes used by early childhood mental health professionals working within primary care settings:

1. When consulting on the psychosocial impact of health conditions,
2. In addressing psychosocial, family, and two-generation factors,
3. While providing prevention, health promotion, and routine well-child visits,
4. Without necessitating a mental health diagnosis as conditional for billing.

Other barriers in traditional healthcare financing models, like limitations on same day or same setting billing by two different providers, would also need to be removed. Beyond FFS options, truly sustainable integrated early childhood behavioral health will likely rely on bundled payment models where early childhood mental health services are packaged within high-quality primary care for children, and capitated/PMPM rates reflect investments in prevention, health promotion, psychosocial screening processes, and interventions.

Acknowledgements Rose Community Foundation, The Colorado Health Foundation, Caring for Colorado Foundation, Walton Family Foundation, Denver Post Season to Share, Roots and Branches of the Rose Community Foundation, and the Irving Harris Foundation generously provided funding for efforts described in this chapter. Healthy Steps for Young Children is supported with funding from the Health Resources and Services Administration and from the Departments of Psychiatry and Pediatrics, University of Colorado School of Medicine. Thank you to our colleagues Lee Savio Beers, M.D., Leandra Godoy, Ph.D., and Sarah Barclay Hoffman at the DC Collaborative for Mental Health in Pediatric Primary Care and New York's Children's Health Home Program for contributing On the Ground examples. We are grateful to the Irving Harris Program in Child Development and Infant Mental Health, the University of Colorado School of Medicine Departments of Pediatrics and Psychiatry, Children's Hospital Colorado, and the Pediatric Mental Health Institute. Finally, we are grateful to the providers, staff, and families in the Child Health Clinic at Children's Hospital Colorado and our Project CLIMB team members for their contributions and ongoing support.

References

Ader, J., Stille, C. J., Keller, D., Miller, B. F., Barr, M. S., & Perrin, J. M. (2015). The medical home and integrated behavioral health: Advancing the policy agenda. *Pediatrics, 135*(5), 909–917.

American Academy of Child and Adolescent Psychiatry Committee on Health Care Access and Economics, American Academy of Pediatrics Task Force on Mental Health. (2009). Improving mental health services in primary care: Reducing administrative and financial barriers to access and collaboration. *Pediatrics, 123*(4), 1248–1251.

American Academy of Pediatrics. (2011). Accountable care organizations (ACOs) and pediatricians: Evaluation and engagement. *AAP News, 32*(1). Retrieved from http://aapnews.aappublications.org/cgi/content/full/32/1/1-e.

American Association of Community Psychiatrists. (2002). *Interface and integration with primary care providers (position paper)*. Dallas, TX: Author. Retrieved from http://www.communitypsychiatry.org/assets/docs/publications/position_statements/ddc-dde.pdf.

American Psychiatric Association. (2002). *Position statement on carve-outs and discrimination.* Retrieved from http://www.psychiatry.org/File%20Library/Advocacy%20and%20Newsroom/Position%20Statements/ps2002_Carve-Outs.pdf.

American Psychological Association. (2004). *Health and behavior* CPT® *codes.* Retrieved from http://www.apapracticecentral.org/reimbursement/billing/secure/new-codes.aspx.

Barlow, J., Wright, C., Sheasby, J., Turner, A., & Hainsworth, J. (2002). Self-management approaches for people with chronic conditions: A review. *Patient Education and Counseling, 48*(2), 177–187.

Barth, M. (2010). Healthy Steps at 15: The past and future of an innovative preventative care model for young children. The Commonwealth Fund. Retrieved from http://www.commonwealthfund.org/content/Publications/Fund-Reports/2010/Dec/Healthy-Steps-at-15.aspx.

Berry, C. A., Krutz, G. S., Langner, B. E., et al. (2008). Jump-starting collaboration: The ABCD initiative and the provision of child development services through Medicaid and collaborators. *Public Administration Review, 68*(3), 480–490.

Briggs, R. D., Stettler, E. M., Silver, E. J., Schrag, R. D., Nayak, M., Chinitz, S. & Racine, A. D. (2012). Social-emotional screening for infants and toddlers in primary care. *Pediatrics, 129*(2), 377–384.

Buchholz, M., Dunn, D., & Badwan, O. (2012, May). *Supporting standardized developmental screening in pediatric primary care: Integrated Mental Health clinicians make a difference.* Poser presentation at the 2012 Developmental Psychobiology Research Group (DPRG) annual retreat, Golden, CO.

Buchholz, M., & Talmi, A. (2012). What we talked about at the pediatrician's office: Exploring differences between Healthy Steps and traditional primary care visits. *Infant Mental Health Journal, 33*(3), 1–7.

Bunik, M., Dunn, D. M., Watkins, L., & Talmi, A. (2014). Trifecta approach to breastfeeding: Clinical care in the integrated mental health model. *Journal of Human Lactation, 30*(2), 143–147. PMID: 24595703.

Bunik, M., & Talmi, A. (2012). *Creating medical homes: Integrating behavioral health services into a residency training pediatric primary care clinic.* MedEdPortal, iCollaborative. Retrieved from https://www.mededportal.org/icollaborative/resource/553.

Chesney, M. L., & Lindeke, L. L. (2012). Accountable care organizations: Advocating for children and PNPs within new models of care. *Journal of Pediatric Health Care, 26*, 312–316.

Cohen, D. J., Davis, M. M., Hall, J. D., Gilchrist, E. C., & Miller, B. F. (2015). *A guidebook of professional practices for behavioral health and primary care integration: Observations from exemplary sites.* Rockville, MD: Agency for Healthcare Research and Quality.

Committee on Child Health Financing. (2013). Medicaid policy statement. *Pediatrics, 131*(5), 1–10.

Current Procedural Terminology (CPT®) copyright 2014. American Medical Association. All rights reserved.

Drotar, D. (2012). Introduction to the special section: Pediatric psychologists' experiences obtaining reimbursement for the use of health and behavior codes. *Journal of Pediatric Psychology, 37*(5), 479–485.

Fisher, E. S., & Shortell, S. M. (2010). Accountable care organizations: Accountable for what, to whom, and how. *Journal of the American Medical Association, 304*(15), 1715–1716.

Golden, O., & Fortuny, K. (2011). *Improving the lives of young children: Meeting parents' health and mental health needs through Medicaid and CHIP so children can thrive.* Washington, DC: The Urban Institute.

Halfon, N., Stevens, G. D., Larson, K., & Olson, L. M. (2011). Duration of a well-child visit: Association with content, family-centeredness, and satisfaction. *Pediatrics, 128*(4), 657–664.

Health Team Works. (2014). Pregnancy related depression symptoms guidance. Retrieved from http://www.healthteamworks.org/guidelines/prd.html

Kaiser Commission on Medicaid and the Uninsured. (2011). A profile of Medicaid managed care programs in 2010: Findings from a 50-state survey. Retrieved from http://kff.org/medicaid/report/a-profile-of-medicaid-managed-care-programs-in-2010-findings-from-a-50-state-survey/

Kathol, R. G., Butler, M., McAlpine, D. D., & Kane, R. L. (2010). Barriers to physical and mental condition integrated service delivery. *Psychosomatic Medicine, 72*(6), 511–518.

Kathol, R. G., Degruy, F., & Rollman, B. L. (2014). Value-based financially sustainable behavioral health components in patient-centered medical homes. *Annals of Family Medicine, 12*(2), 172–175.

Kelleher, K. J., & Stevens, J. (2009). Evolution of child mental health services in primary care. *Academic Pediatrics, 9*(1), 7–14.

King, T. M., Tandon, S. D., Macias, M. M., Healy, J. A., Duncan, P. M., Swigonski, N. L., … Lipkin, P. H. (2010). Implementing developmental screening and referrals: Lessons learned from a national project. *Pediatrics, 125*(2), 350–360.

Lewis, V. A., Colla, C. H., Tierney, K., Van Citters, A. D., Fisher, E. S., & Meara, E. (2014). Few ACOs pursue innovative models that integrate care for mental illness and substance abuse with primary care. *Health Affairs, 33*(10), 1808–1816.

Lines, M. M., Tynan, W. D., Angalet, G. B., & Pendley, J. S. (2012). Commentary: The use of health and behavior codes in pediatric psychology: Where are we now? *Journal of Pediatric Psychology, 37*(5), 486–490.

Lovell, J. L., Roemer, R., & Talmi, A. (2014, May). Pregnancy-related depression screening and services in pediatric primary care. *CYF Newsletter of the American Psychological Association.* Retrieved from: http://www.apa.org/pi/families/resources/newsletter/2014/05/pregnancy-depression.aspx

Mauch, D. (2002). Managed care in the public sector. In D. Feldman (Ed.), *Managed behavioral health services: Perspectives and practice.* Springfield, IL: Charles C Thomas.

Mauch, D., Kautz, C., & Smith, S. A. (2008). *Reimbursement of mental health services in primary care settings (HHS Pub. No. SMA-08-4324).* Rockville, MD: Center for Mental Health Services, Substance Abuse and Mental Health Services Administration.

Miller, H. (2009). From volume to value: Better ways to pay for health care. *Health Affairs, 28,* 1418–1428.

Minkovitz, C. S., Strobino, D., Mistry, K. B., Scharfstein, D. O., Grason, H., Hou, W., … Guyer, B. (2007). Healthy Steps for Young Children: Sustained results at 5.5 years. *Pediatrics, 120*(3), 658–668.

Monson, S. P., Sheldon, J. C., Ivey, L. C., Kinman, C. R., & Beacham, A. O. (2012). Working toward financial sustainability of integrated behavioral health services in a public health care system. *Families, Systems & Health, 30*(2), 181–186.

Murray, L., Fearon, P., & Cooper, P. (2015). Postnatal depression, mother-infant interactions, and child development. In J. Milgrom & A. Gemmill (Eds.), *Identifying perinatal depression and anxiety: Evidenced-based practice in screening, psychosocial assessment, and management* (pp. 139–164). Malden, MA: Wiley-Blackwell.

National Academy for State Health Policy. (2009). About ABCD. Retrieved from http://www.nashp.org/abcd-history

National Committee for Quality Assurance. (2010). Accountable care organizations (ACO) draft 2011 criteria. Retrieved from http://www.ncqa.org/portals/0/publiccomment/ACO/ACO_%20Overview.pdf

Patient Protection and Affordable Care Act, 42 U.S.C. § 18001 (2010).

Radecki, L., Sand-Loud, N., O'Connor, K. G., Sharp, S., & Olson, L. M. (2011). Trends in the use of standardized tools for developmental screening in early childhood: 2002-2009. *Pediatrics, 128*(1), 14–19.

Rosenberg, S. A., Zhang, D., & Robinson, C. C. (2008). Prevalence of developmental delays and participation in early intervention services for young children. *Pediatrics, 121*(6), e1503–e1509.

Rosenthal, T. C. (2008). The medical home: Growing evidence to support a new approach to primary care. *Journal of the American Board of Family Medicine, 21*(5), 427–440.

Selker, H. P., Kravitz, R. L., & Gallagher, T. H. (2014). The national physician payment commission recommendation to eliminate fee-for-service payment: Balancing risk, benefit, and efficiency in bundling payment for care. *Journal of General Internal Medicine, 29*(5), 698–699.

Summer, L., & Hoadley, J. (2014). *The role of Medicaid managed care in health delivery system innovation.* New York: The Commonwealth Fund. Retrieved from http://www.commonwealthfund.org/~/media/files/publications/fund-report/2014/apr/1741_summer_role_medicaid:managed_care_hlt_sys_delivery.pdf

Swartz, M., & Morrissey, J. (2012). Health center reimbursement for behavioral health services in Medicaid: National Association of Community Health Centers, 2010. *North Carolina Medical Journal, 73*, 177–184.

Talmi, A., Bunik, M., Asherin, R., Rannie, M., Watlington, T., Beaty, B., & Berman, S. (2014). Improving developmental screening documentation and referral completion. *Pediatrics, 134*(4), e1181–e1188. (PMID: 25180272).

Talmi, A., & Fazio, E. (2012). Commentary: Promoting health and well-being in pediatric primary care settings: Using health and behavior codes at routine well-child visits. *Journal of Pediatric Psychology, 37*(5), 496–502.

Talmi, A., Stafford, B., & Buchholz, M. (2009). Perinatal mental health where the babies are, in pediatric primary care. *Zero to Three, 29*(5), 10–16.

Chapter 10
Considerations for Planning and Conducting an Evaluation

Ellen Johnson Silver and Rosy Chhabra

Abstract Upon embarking upon integrated early childhood behavioral health programming, consideration of evaluation processes and specification of expected and desired outcomes are essential. Needs for evaluative data are quite diverse, depending on the varied expectations of stakeholders. Just as there are numerous reasons why one needs to evaluate, there are many different methods that can be used. Designing an evaluation involves a number of important considerations (e.g., deciding when to start and when to finish, what information to collect, and what data collection methods might work best for the population being studied) and there is no one approach that works best in all instances. A key question to ask when deciding on an approach is whether the evaluation design is strong enough to produce trustworthy evidence that the program or intervention works. In sum, the value of evaluation is frequently minimized. Because of this it is often overlooked and many times is the last component of planning, but it should be a key component from the start of any process, project, or program. This chapter discusses reasons why evaluations can and should be done, some considerations for developing an evaluation focus, and elements of evaluation, including measures. It concludes with an evaluation example from the field of integrated early childhood behavioral health programs, which describes the design and results of a parent experiences and satisfaction survey used to assess the effectiveness of Healthy Steps at Montefiore.

Keyword Evaluation • Assessment • Data

Introduction

Evaluation is an essential practice that is systematically designed and instituted to establish the significance of a process, project, and/or program. It also provides a basis for understanding the value of a system or an organization from a broader

E.J. Silver, Ph.D. (✉) • R. Chhabra, Psy.D.
Albert Einstein College of Medicine, Bronx, NY, USA
e-mail: ellen.silver@einstein.yu.edu; rosy.chhabra@einstein.yu.edu

© Springer International Publishing Switzerland 2016   165
R.D. Briggs (ed.), *Integrated Early Childhood Behavioral Health in Primary Care*, DOI 10.1007/978-3-319-31815-8_10

perspective. The decisions behind any evaluation, which include defining its need and including it in the design of a program, are sometimes misunderstood and the inherent value that an evaluation can provide is often minimized. While evaluation is often overlooked and many times is the last component of planning, it should be a key component from the start to plan a systematic process to identify information and data that need to be collected in order to demonstrate successful outcomes or efficacy. In this chapter, we discuss some of the ways evaluation is important and how it might proceed depending on its purpose and intended audience.

There are several reasons why one needs to evaluate as there can be many different users of the evaluation results whose needs for evaluative data are quite diverse. For example, there is increasing emphasis on the use of evidence-based practice and evidence-based interventions throughout the fields of medicine, psychology, and public health, and on gathering the best available research evidence on whether and why a program works and for whom. Data derived through systematic evaluation can help assess the utility of a program or initiative and determine whether a program should be continued or terminated, or if it can be improved or expanded. Many of those who are intended users of the evaluation findings are management level roles who will need data to inform the decision-making process. How they take action related to a program or initiative can therefore be very dependent on evaluation findings, interpretation of results, and the types of recommendations made. Program evaluations are also frequently obtained in order to satisfy the needs for accountability presented by program funders and sponsors who want to assure that their money is well-spent (Rossi, Lipsey, & Freeman, 2004). Others who rely on evaluation results might be government agencies making decisions about funding, or policy or community organizations deciding what programs to advocate for with these agencies. Other users of evaluation findings may be those directly involved with a program, such as clients who want credible and useful information to guide their selection of a program, or the community groups who serve them and desire advice and direction on which programs to support and recommend. Finally, evaluation research may contribute to fundamental social science knowledge (Rossi et al., 2004). Evaluations, like other types of research, can provide data that test theoretical models about how to bring about change and are of value to the scientific and academic community.

A key question to ask when deciding on an evaluation approach is whether the design is strong enough to produce trustworthy evidence that the program or intervention works (NFECPE, 2007), and it has been suggested that one important facet of good enough evaluation is that it be systematic and follow a set of logical rules and procedures (Rossi et al., 2004). Rossi et al. (2004) provide a comprehensive picture of the competing demands that sometimes arise between viewing the purpose of evaluation research as meeting demands of decision makers and stakeholders and the pragmatics of striving to meet exacting scientific standards. They suggest that while both are important, they are not always compatible. Not all designs that look best from a scientific standpoint are feasible in a "real-life" context. Importantly, the levels of expertise and resources needed to produce evaluations that conform to the scientific ideal are often not achievable, and in practice a balance must be found between use of methods and procedures that safeguard validity of findings without jeopardizing the need to make them timely, meaningful, and useful.

In general, to evaluate a program's outcomes, one will ask how much change it brought about in desired outcomes and whether there are things one might do to improve its efficacy. But some programs are more effective for some subgroups of participants than they are for others. Thus, another important aspect of any evaluation would be to determine whether the characteristics of those who do and do not achieve the desired outcomes differ in any measurable way. These types of data help us to target interventions and determine whether they meet the needs of identified population. In an evaluation, one also needs to understand dosage, i.e., how much of the intervention is needed to get to the desired levels of the outcomes and whether there are important differences in outcomes based on how many program activities or sessions were completed. These considerations may be particularly relevant regarding integrated early childhood behavioral health programs, which often provide variable levels of service based on need, as they care for large, heterogeneous groups of patients.

Considerations for Developing an Evaluation Focus

Designing an evaluation involves many considerations. In simple terms, the context, content, design, and impact of any evaluation are based on the needs of the main stakeholders for the evaluation, the reason or purpose for conducting an evaluation, and the decisions that need to be made as a result of the evaluation's findings (Coombes, 2009; Habicht, Victora, & Vaughan, 1999; McNamara, 2005). We have identified four important considerations: defining the purpose, identifying the audience, measurement decisions, and deciding the timing of the evaluation.

1. *Defining the purpose of the evaluation*: Why do we need to do this evaluation? What do we need to find out? The purpose of any evaluation is usually to answer specific questions, such as addressing program quality, implementation, and effectiveness. The purpose of the evaluation not only informs the large-scale evaluation design, but also directs the variables involved in the evaluation (e.g., stakeholder focus, accountability, time limits, available resources, and type of evaluation). For example, the main highlights of conducting a community program evaluation might include sharing the benefits of the program with the community, organization, or funder; developing and maintaining the focus of the work being done; and breaking down the components of the program to understand how, what, and why any aspect is useful, and for whom.
2. *Identifying the evaluation audience*: Who are the stakeholders who require the evaluation? How does it need to be presented? Each different type of stakeholder might require that information be shared in a specific way that is useful to them. For example, the evaluation and the presentation would differ if one is conducting the evaluation to share with researchers, specific population groups, funders,

organizational supervisors, and/or the general population. If the evaluation is for the research community, the findings could be a published manuscript in a journal, or could be shared as a presentation at a conference. If the evaluation is about efficacy of a certain program at the personnel level, the report might be developed for a management level presentation and focus on ways to improve that program. Alternatively, it could focus on creating a feedback system to adapt or transform the program to be more effective. If one is investigating health-related outcomes, an evaluation might adapt the Triple Aim framework (Berwick, Nolan, & Whittington, 2008) and look towards improving the health of the patient population, improving the experience of the care system, and reducing care costs. Each of these possibilities would lead to different evaluation questions, data sources, data collection techniques, analytic strategies, and presentation formats.

3. *Deciding how to measure success or effectiveness*: It is important to identify and determine the key outcomes, activities, and markers required for evaluation during the planning stages of any project. Outcomes usually refer to what one wants to accomplish in terms of effectiveness or impact. Activities are more about what to do in the process of reaching those outcomes in terms of the interventions that will be given to participants. Markers/indicators demonstrate what progress is being made in the quality and quantity of the activities being delivered (Boulmetis & Dutwin, 2005; Gajda & Jewiss, 2004). Some of the important components to be considered are:

   (a) What questions need to be answered in the evaluation? These are defined as what the stakeholders need to know in order to make an informed decision about a project or program. The sources of data could be existing records/information or might require measures to collect new data. For example, if one needs information about how teenage pregnancy has changed over the years in a community in order to plan a pregnancy prevention initiative, one could look at the existing data sources from the city, county, or state where this kind of information is collected and do a secondary analysis of the data to get the information. On the other hand, if one wants to find out whether an intervention will make a difference in the rates of teenage pregnancy in a particular school or region, one would need to evaluate a specific intervention with outcome measures that are culturally and developmentally appropriate for the teenage population of that school or region.

   (b) What kind of information needs to be collected in order to answer the key questions about the program? The depth of inquiry and measures used are grounded in the purpose and the audience identified. For example, does one need to collect demographics of a population and specific measures of outcomes to evaluate the efficacy of a program for a specific population, or does one need to collect information regarding the organizational structure of an institution to assess the availability of funding to conduct the program for that population (also known as "defining the purpose")? Is the information collected going to be shared with the community and/or be published in a journal and/or does the funder need the information in order to understand organizational capacity to conduct a specified program ("defining the audience")?

(c) How are the data being collected? Decisions about the best way to collect the data are often predicated on the framework one utilizes for the evaluation. For example, if one needs to decide which issues are affecting a community in order to design a specific program for that community, one might conduct focus groups and/or individual interviews (e.g., qualitative data collection) with the key stakeholders in the community to identify main issues of concern, and design the intervention accordingly. However, if one is trying to evaluate the success of a program based on specific constructs, one might use measures that evaluate those constructs to collect information from the participants (e.g., quantitative data collection) before and after the program or intervention. For example, if the intervention is designed to increase a participant's emotional well-being, then the outcome measures would likely focus on psychological distress symptoms or on quality of life.

(d) What is the timeline? Will participants answer the evaluation measures only once (meaning one data collection point) or do they need to be followed for a period of time (i.e., more than one data collection point) to determine whether there are lasting changes or to uncover new impacts that emerge at later times? Will there need to be baseline data collection, before a program is implemented? There are different issues to consider if one is evaluating a program that requires one time data collection directly after an intervention versus follow-up for a longer period of time. One must determine the optimal number of time points, how to account for potential loss of data over time, and the possibility of historical or developmental changes, especially relevant within the highly variable early childhood period.

4. *Deciding when to conduct the evaluation*: Evaluation is not a set process that has to happen at a certain time or only in a particular way. Many times an evaluation is conducted at the beginning (while one is writing the proposal to identify gaps or the areas of importance for the study/intervention, often referred to as a needs assessment), during the study or program (a process evaluation of how well and why some components are working or not working), before the end of the study to understand if it is working as intended (to find out if the study was successful in reaching some of its short-term goals) and finally after the study is completed to assess the outcomes and impact.

Types of Evaluation

A useful way to describe evaluation for all of the above mentioned issues is in terms of formative and summative evaluations. Formative evaluations usually entail an ongoing process, possibly starting from defining the issue and development of the study content and then continuing to assess whether the direction of the program/ study is moving in the expected direction and is doing so within the given time frame. There are several types of formative evaluations, such as (a) Needs Assessment—defining the level and extent of the issues/problem, determining how the identified population is being affected and what has already been tried and tested; (b) Evaluation ability and feasibility—asking whether the identified issues or problems can be specified and evaluated. This effort may also take the perspectives of the affected community into consideration; (c) Program and outcome conceptualization—whether the population and/or the stakeholders can define the needed program constructs and the suggested outcomes; and (d) Implementation and Process Evaluation—monitoring whether the program is being delivered accurately and reliably as well as describing as the process of delivery.

In contrast, summative evaluation is usually completed at the end of the program and basically collects information about whether aims and/or objectives of a study/program have been met. Types of summative evaluations include: (a) Impact evaluation—assessing if the program had the intended or different effects and (b) Outcome evaluation—determining if the program was able to provide defined changes or effects on an identified population. Other types of summative evaluations identified in the literature include conducting cost-benefit and/or effectiveness evaluations (see more about cost-benefit analyses in Chap. 3 of this volume by Racine); secondary analysis to utilize existing data to address new effects/areas and/or to utilize new statistical techniques; and integrating data from various studies to conduct meta-analysis in order to answer more general population-level evaluation questions (Boulmetis & Dutwin, 2011).

Designing an Evaluation

Outcome Evaluation Overview Many methods can be used in outcome evaluation and there is no single design that works best in all circumstances. As each method is likely to have some limitations and biases, a combination of approaches and perspectives often works best. Many of the approaches utilized in evaluation come from methods developed in the social sciences and they may include experimental, quasi-experimental, and other less traditional designs (CDC, 1999; NREPP, 2012; Rossi et al., 2004).

Experimental Designs The experimental design or randomized controlled trial (RCT) is generally thought of as the strongest design and the gold standard for research (CDC, 1999). This is because it allows a comparison of outcomes for people that receive the intervention or services ("experimental group") to those of an otherwise equivalent group of people who do not ("control group"). The control group may receive something else instead of the intervention, which could be another program or "standard care," or they may receive nothing at all. The key aspect of this design is the random assignment to groups, which increases the likelihood that the characteristics and attitudes of the people in the experimental group and the control group will be the same before the intervention takes place. Without randomization, it is likely that there will be selection bias, as the people who decide to attend the program being evaluated could be different from those who don't enroll in ways that influence the outcomes of interest. Because randomization creates two groups that would be similar if not for the intervention, we can be fairly confident that any differences in outcomes between the two groups following the program can be attributed to its effects and not to some other thing (NFECPE, 2007; NREPP, 2012; Tebes, Kaufman, & Connell, 2003). However, randomization does not guarantee that there will be no important group differences that can affect outcomes, and when looking at effects the evaluator must check for preexisting differences in characteristics and ensure that the groups are actually comparable at baseline (NREPP, 2012). If they are not, then appropriate statistical controls often can and should be applied. It is also critical to determine whether comparable alternative programs and services were available to those in the control group. If the control group's members are able to seek out and receive an intervention similar to the one being evaluated, the contrast between the groups may be small and the program may appear less effective than it really is (NFECPE, 2007).

Quasi-Experimental Designs In some circumstances, trying to conduct a RCT is not a reasonable approach to determine whether an intervention has the desired impact, but there may be alternative ways of constructing "no treatment" groups that are similar to the experimental group (NFECPE, 2007). Quasi-experimental methods are not considered to have a true control condition because the study groups are preexisting or self-selected rather than created through random assignment, and the researcher is not the one who manipulates the "exposure" variable (i.e., who does or does not get the program). For example, an administrator in a pediatric primary care setting might be unwilling to allow individuals to be randomly assigned to experimental and control groups due to ethical concerns, as he or she believes it would deny treatment to those who need it (NREPP, 2012). In such cases, the evaluator will sometimes compare program participants to those on a waiting list or to community members matched on important characteristics to the participants. Another approach would be to compare similarly matched individuals in communities with and without the program (CDC, 1999). The disadvantage to quasi-experimental designs is that it is not possible to make definitive causal inferences about the impact of the intervention. However, quasi-experimental designs also have advantages. Because they share many of the same elements as RCTs, these designs provide an opportunity to systematically evaluate outcomes (when an experimental design is not practical) and thus can be an excellent option for small programs that either lack resources to run a full-scale RCT or programs who cannot randomize participation. As previously noted, a key consideration is making sure that the groups are equivalent and, if needed, to employ statistical controls when analyzing outcomes.

Other Designs In some instances, other less traditional designs such as simple before and after (pretest and posttest) or posttest-only designs may be suitable for measuring progress toward achieving desired program goals (CDC, 1999). These designs are defined by lack of random assignment as well as the absence of a control or comparison condition, as only the program participants are tracked (NREPP, 2012), so it is even more difficult to rule out alternate explanations for post-intervention outcomes and attribute causality. A pretest and posttest design measures outcomes among program participants before and after the intervention, whereas in the post-test-only design, outcome data are collected from participants only after the program's completion (NREPP, 2012). The major drawback of a posttest-only evaluation is that it does not address change as there is no baseline measure to which post-intervention results can be compared. Occasionally, when using a posttest design, the evaluator also asks participants to report on their behavior or attitudes prior to the program in addition to asking them about their current status, but of course these perceptions or attributions can be subject to distortions and recall bias.

Observational or nonexperimental designs are other types of designs often used in traditional evaluations and include cross-sectional surveys, time series, and case studies, among others. Periodic cross-sectional surveys of selected community samples can inform your evaluation (CDC, 1999), but there is no natural ordering of the observations. In time series, on the other hand, the sequencing and intervals among the data points over a specific time period is meaningful and yields its own statistics. It can provide data on trends, patterns, and turning points. Although case studies may utilize quantitative, qualitative, or mixed methods to collect information, they tend to be more qualitative in nature and provide an in-depth understanding of the "whys" and "hows" of an intervention, population, process, program, or system within a given context. This approach highlights the context as it tries to explore and explain causal associations, but a significant limitation is that results may be hard to generalize to other contexts and situations (Sartorius et al., 2013).

Administrative Evaluations Another important aspect of evaluation relates to administrative evaluation and this is often focused on the feasibility and fidelity of delivering a program. In terms of feasibility, we may want to know whether the program was successful in reaching the people for whom it was intended. Thus, we might wish to assess recruitment and retention. It is helpful to know whether the intended targets of an intervention are familiar with it, whether they decide to participate and actually enroll in the program, and whether they stay in it long enough to benefit from the activities. Part of the administrative evaluation might determine who decides to participate and who does not, or who drops out and when, i.e., what are the characteristics of these different groups and how do they influence recruitment and retention? We also might ask what barriers to participation they encountered so that we can modify the program for future groups. Evaluating fidelity is also critical because it assesses whether the essential elements or components of the program were delivered as planned. This may be measured both in terms of the amount of intervention that was expected to be provided to participants, and whether the people delivering the program were proficient in doing so according to the specific guidelines of the program. If a program is not successful in achieving outcomes, there is no way to tell whether this reflects a failure of the underlying theoretical model, or, on the other hand, failure to implement the model as intended unless adherence to the expected activities and procedures is well monitored. Thus, use of valid fidelity criteria is an expected part of quality program evaluation practice (Mowbray, Holter, Teague, & Bybee, 2003).

An additional area of administrative evaluation involves assessing participants' satisfaction with the quality of the program and how well the program meets their needs, either overall or in terms of its different components. Depending on the program's goals and objectives, we may assess whether participants felt helped by the program or if it increased their knowledge in some way. We also might collect other types of feedback and ask about things that made them like or dislike the program, and these could have little or nothing to do with its effectiveness in terms of our intended outcomes.

Many evaluations also consider financial aspects of a program. Cost is often a critical factor in deciding whether to maintain or terminate a program. Cost analysis on its own involves determining all of the costs associated with an intervention (Preskill & Russ-Eft, 2005). However, what is commonly measured and of greater concern are estimates of cost-effectiveness or cost-benefits (Preskill & Russ-Eft, 2005; Tebes et al., 2003). In both cost-effectiveness and cost-benefits evaluations, the costs are measured in dollars or some other monetary unit (Preskill & Russ-Eft, 2005). In a cost-effectiveness evaluation, the effectiveness measure may include outcomes such as new skills competencies or improved satisfaction (Tebes et al., 2003). A cost-benefit analysis transforms the effects or results of a program into dollars or some other monetary unit, and the costs are then compared to the benefits using the same unit of measurement (Tebes et al., 2003). The decision maker must decide whether the costs justify the outcomes. Unfortunately, estimating costs is quite complex. It is often difficult to know what standard or perspective to consider in deciding if the cost is reasonable in relation to benefits of achieving your program's goals and objectives, or to know whether all of the important costs and benefits have been included in one's estimates (Tebes et al., 2003). Please see Chap. 3 by Racine in this volume for more information on this subject.

Finally, another aspect of an administrative evaluation is the issue of sustainability. Discussions and use of survey tools with sponsors, partners, and other stakeholders about their organizational willingness and capacity, financial and otherwise, to assure the program can continue and maintain its benefits to participants over the long term can be of great value. When assessing sustainability of a program, the data from many other parts of the evaluation are likely to contribute to the endeavor.

Selecting Measures

Gathering evidence of the effectiveness, fidelity, feasibility, or costs of a program can involve a range of tools and measures. The data collected for the evaluation might be quantitative and include surveys or ratings or even measures of attendance and other results that can be shared numerically. Qualitative assessments may include focus groups or narratives and utilize observational and verbal descriptions to share results. Mixed methods evaluation intentionally combines both quantitative and qualitative data in order to draw upon the strengths of each method. Data may be gathered from participants, from providers or other interventionists, through observations or video/audiotaping of program activities or through reviews of administrative/program documents and records. Use of multiple sources and types of data collection methods are useful in improving accuracy of evaluations because they look at the outcomes from various angles and may reveal different things about the various components of the program. Just as with any other type of research, it is important to consider whether the instruments chosen and procedures for administering them are valid for capturing the information needed in the particular community being evaluated. Any flaws in the instruments used or inconsistencies in how they are administered can skew results (NREPP, 2012), so it is very important to know the norming population for any scales that are employed, and the official guidelines for administration. In most cases, especially where measures have not been validated in a specific group, it would be beneficial to conduct pilot testing to determine the appropriateness of using the measure with a particular population and to help refine the measure if needed.

Timing of Measurements

The timing of the posttest data collection is important and should allow enough time for the program to have a measurable effect without allowing so much time to pass that effects are diluted or influenced by participation in other programs or by environmental/historical events unrelated to participation (NREPP, 2012). Maturation or the normal processes of development that occur over time also could affect measured outcomes, especially when the participants in the program being evaluated are young children. Depending on timing of posttests, changes could be due to development of new skills or to improvements in existing abilities that emerge as children grow and mature, which occur independently of the specific intervention being tested. Thus, it is important to be aware of any potential competing reasons for changes over time and to note them in evaluation reports as well.

Follow-up measurements over repeated periods can tell you if a program has a sustained effect beyond the immediate treatment period. There are also some circumstances where no immediate effects are found, but later delayed effects emerge. However, it is sometimes difficult and costly to conduct long-term follow-up assessments and procedures for ensuring retention over the follow-up period must be carefully developed (NREPP, 2012). Evaluators should also keep in mind that if the same measures are re-administered multiple times, participants could become bored or annoyed and may be less interested in continuing to complete them. This can affect response rates or how participants answer questions. Administering a measure multiple times can also affect results simply because the participants become familiar with the tool (NREPP, 2012). Because it can be difficult to determine if effects seen over time are caused by the program or the administration of prior tests, these issues must be considered in planning how and when to administer evaluation measures.

Summary

In summary, when embarking upon integrated early childhood behavioral health programming, consideration of evaluation processes and outcomes is essential. In order to evaluate its effectiveness, one first needs to determine the goals and desired outcomes of any identified program and the types of indicators that will assist in determining how much progress, if any, has been made in achieving the desired outcomes. An outcome evaluation investigates whether changes have occurred for the people participating in a program, how big those changes are, and whether they are positive or negative.

On the Ground Example: Evaluation of Healthy Steps at Montefiore—Parent Experiences and Satisfaction

Background In Chap. 5, Kaplan-Sanoff and Briggs reviewed the history and design of Healthy Steps, and in Chap. 7, Briggs, Schrag Hershberg, and Germán describe how it was implemented at our medical center, which included a discussion of modifications over the course of expansion. For the initial research evaluation, Healthy Steps at Montefiore enrolled first-time mothers and their partners, either during the last trimester of pregnancy or before the child was 2 months old. The evaluation involved a periodic longitudinal assessment of the well-being of the children and their mothers who were followed for 36 months when the intervention was completed. This was not a RCT. Instead it was a quasi-experimental study in which Healthy Steps at Montefiore participants were enrolled and assessed in the intervention site and a demographically similar comparison group was recruited from a matched clinical site at our medical center and followed separately in order to determine whether the program was having the anticipated effects.

The primary outcome variable we considered in evaluating our Healthy Steps program was the child's social-emotional status (Briggs et al., 2014). As part of the evaluation of our Healthy Steps program, we used the Ages and Stages Questionnaires: Social-Emotional (ASQ:SE) (Squires, Bricker, & Twombly, 2002) to screen for problems in the child's socioemotional functioning at various intervals up to 36 months of age, which is when participation in the program ended. At the final data collection we assessed 85 Healthy Steps children and 39 from the comparison group. Multiple regression analyses showed that receiving the Healthy Steps program was significantly associated with lower (better) ASQ:SE scores at 36 months. Because we hypothesized that caregiver experiences of childhood trauma would be related to deficits in social-emotional development in their children, we conducted subgroup analyses to see whether participating in Healthy Steps moderated the impact of maternal childhood trauma on their children. We found that while children of mothers with childhood trauma had higher (worse) 36-month ASQ:SE mean scores than children of mothers without childhood trauma overall, participation in Montefiore's Healthy Steps program seemed to moderate this relationship.

In addition to the outcome evaluation, we conducted a survey about parent experiences and satisfaction at child age 36 months. In recent years, there has been increasing interest in and emphasis on patient-centered care including the inclusion of consumer input into decision-making. One arm of the "Triple Aim" statement (Berwick, Nolan, & Whittington, 2008) regarding optimizing healthcare system performance refers to the importance of "improving the patient experience of care," which is held to be equally as important as reducing costs and improving health outcomes. Beyond the obvious intrinsic value, the patient experience of care or patient satisfaction may drive decisions related to choosing one practice over another, demonstrating the important relationship between patient experience and revenue.

The main goal of our parent experiences and satisfaction survey was to understand maternal perceptions of the Healthy Steps at Montefiore program. Healthy Steps is a national program and has demonstrated improved patient satisfaction where it has been implemented (Minkovitz et al., 2007). However, the original research reports for Healthy Steps (Minkovitz et al., 2001) described findings related to quality of care, patient satisfaction, and parenting within a largely Caucasian, middle income population. In contrast, Healthy Steps at Montefiore began in 2006 with a distinctly different patient population, which was largely Hispanic and Black and low income. Thus we sought to see if we would replicate findings related to patient perceptions and satisfaction within our own community.

Measures To conduct this parent satisfaction evaluation, we contacted the original Healthy Steps study authors and acquired copies of the parent satisfaction evaluation they had used, and then integrated the same questions when possible into our own program completion survey, which was administered to both the treatment and comparison group. These included 15 statements about the care received from their child's doctor, to which they indicated how much they agreed or disagreed. There were both positive statements (e.g., the doctor always has time to answer my questions, the doctor points out what I do well as a parent) and negative statements (the doctor seems to have other things on his or her mind when we talk, the doctor acts like I can't understand information about child growth and development). The survey also asked parents whether they would recommend their clinic, if anyone from the clinic visited the home and what that person did, and whether the parent was satisfied with the services that they provided. Parents were also asked about receiving emotional support at the clinic, about parent support groups, classes or other events for parents they may have attended, about referrals for the child that they received, and whether anyone at the clinic talked to them about relevant child development topics (e.g., toilet training, language development, home safety).

Procedures To maintain privacy and confidentiality, the program completion survey at the intervention site was self-administered. It was handed out by the front desk staff and parents were asked to complete it at any time during their child's 36-month visit. Parents were requested to place the completed evaluation in a manila envelope, seal it, and place it in a protected mailbox for retrieval by the Program Director. For the comparison group, surveys were administered by a research assistant in the waiting room of the practice.

Results There were 89 Healthy Steps at Montefiore parents and 48 comparison group parents who participated in the outcome evaluation that was done at 36 months. Of these, 52 Healthy Steps participants and 39 comparison group parents responded to the program completion survey. Results of this evaluation showed that parents in Healthy Steps at Montefiore were significantly more likely to say they would recommend their clinic to a friend or family member (100 % vs. 89 %; $p < .04$). They also were more likely to report that they had received needed emotional support to cope with stress through the clinic (75 % vs. 43 %, $p < .04$) and that they had attended any parent support groups or parenting related events (42 % vs. 5 %, $p < .0001$). More Healthy Steps parents also said that their child had been referred to testing for concerns about progress in walking, talking, or hearing (30 % vs. 11 %, $p < .03$). Parents enrolled in Healthy Steps were more likely to say they had talked to someone or received information about the importance of regular routines for young children (94 % vs. 65 %, $p < .0001$); child language development (92 % vs. 62 %, $p < .001$); toilet training (90 % vs. 64 %, $p < .01$); home safety (92 % vs. 76 %, $p < .03$); child development (98 % vs. 78 %, $p < .01$); child temperament (94 % vs. 68 %; $p < .001$); sleep problems (84 % vs. 60 %, $p < .01$); and discipline (96 % vs. 60 %, $p < .0001$). Although the trends were in the same direction, Healthy Steps parents did not differ significantly from comparison group in talking about or receiving information on sibling rivalry (51 % vs. 40 %) and ways to help children learn (90 % vs. 78 %). Many more Healthy Steps parents said they had received a home visit (59 % vs. 3 %, $p < .0001$); because only one comparison group parent had done so, we could not compare satisfaction with these services by group. The two groups of parents did not differ in any of the 15 items asking about care that their children received from their primary care providers; most parents, irrespective of the practice site they attended with their children, agreed or strongly agreed with positive statements and disagreed or strongly agreed with negative ones.

Discussion The results described above both support and compliment the findings of the outcome evaluation looking at child social-emotional functioning (Briggs et al., 2014). Caregiver reports about their experiences in Healthy Steps at Montefiore provided evidence related to fidelity as they showed that, as planned, they received supportive services beyond the usual standard of care. It also helped establish that the comparison group did not receive services from their primary care clinic or elsewhere that were comparable to those received by participating Healthy Steps families. If this occurred, it might have compromised our ability to find group differences in outcomes (NFECPE, 2007). We also showed that the Healthy Steps parents found these services helpful and that parents in the two groups were equally satisfied with their medical providers. This latter finding was not unexpected as the practices, while in separate buildings in different neighborhoods, treated very similar patient populations and shared many characteristics, including being in the same division of the pediatrics department, having the same medical director, and having comparable staffing levels (Briggs et al., 2014). Moreover, it also helped to verify that we selected an appropriate comparison group for the evaluation. However, there are some limitations of this evaluation, the most important of which is a high attrition rate. As far as we could ascertain, this was primarily due to families either moving out of the area or choosing to go to other providers closer to their homes. Because our practice site also houses the high-risk obstetrics and gynecology practice for the borough, families with newborns frequently begin their pediatric care there, but then move to a more geographically convenient practice later. Nevertheless we cannot be sure whether the parents who left from the two sites were different in their use of or satisfaction with services, which could affect this comparison.

Final Thoughts

The above description of the Healthy Steps at Montefiore parent satisfaction survey is just one example of an early childhood integrated behavioral health evaluation protocol. We hope that this chapter has presented a helpful framework for considering evaluation design questions, and strongly encourage those in the field to incorporate evaluation into their planning from the inception.

References

Berwick, D. M., Nolan, T. W., & Whittington, J. (2008). The triple aim: Care, health and cost. *Health Affairs, 27*, 759–769.

Boulmetis, J., & Dutwin, P. (2005). *The ABCs of evaluation: Timeless techniques for program and project managers* (2nd ed.). San Francisco, CA: Jossey-Bass.

Boulmetis, J., & Dutwin, P. (2011). *The ABCs of evaluation: Timeless techniques for program and project managers* (3rd ed.). San Francisco, CA: Jossey-Bass.

Briggs, R., Silver, E. J., Krug, L. M., Mason, Z. S., Schrag, R. D. A., Chinitz, S. P., Racine, A. D. (2014). Health steps as a moderator: The impact of maternal trauma on child social-emotional development. *Clinical Practice in Pediatric Psychology, 2*, 166–175.

CDC. (1999). *Framework for program evaluation in public health*. Atlanta, GA: Center for Disease Control and Prevention.

Coombes, Y. (2009). Evaluating according to purpose and resources. In M. Thorogood & Y. Coombes (Eds.), *Evaluating health promotion: Practice and methods*. Oxford, England: Oxford University Press (Oxford Scholarship Online).

Gajda, R., & Jewiss, J. (2004). Thinking about how to evaluate your program? These strategies will get you started [Electronic Version]. *Practical assessment, research & evaluation, 9*. Retrieved September 25, 2015 from http://pareonline.net/getvn.asp?v=9&n=8

Habicht, J. P., Victora, C. G., & Vaughan, J. P. (1999). Evaluation designs for adequacy, plausibility and probability of public health programme performance and impact. *International Journal of Epidemiology, 28*(1), 10–18.

McNamara, C. (2005). *Field guide to consulting and organizational development: A collaborative and systems approach to performance, change and learning*. Minneapolis, MN: Authenticity Consulting LLC.

Minkovitz, C., Strobino, D., Hughart, N., Scharfstein, D., Guyer, B., & Healthy Steps Evaluation Team. (2001). Early effects of the healthy steps for young children program. *Archives of Pediatrics and Adolescent Medicine, 155*(4), 470–479.

Minkovitz, C. S., Strobino, D., Mistry, K. B., Scharfstein, D. O., Grason, H., Hou, W., … Guyer, B. (2007). Healthy steps for young children: Sustained results at 5.5 years. *Pediatrics, 120*(3), e658–e668.

Mowbray, C. T., Holter, M. C., Teague, G. B., & Bybee, D. (2003). Fidelity criteria: Development, measurement, and validation. *American Journal of Evaluation, 24*(3), 315–340.

NFECPE. (2007). *Early childhood program evaluations: A decision-makers guide*. Center on Developing Child at Harvard University: National Forum on Early Childhood Program Evaluations.

NREPP. (2012). Non-researcher's guide to evidence-based program evaluation. Retrieved August 31, 2015 from http://nrepp.samhsa.gov/Courses/ProgramEvaluation/NREPP_0401_0010.html.

Preskill, H., & Russ-Eft, D. (2005). *Building evaluation capacity: 72 activities for teaching and training*. Thousand Oaks, CA: Sage.

Rossi, P. H., Lipsey, M. W., & Freeman, H. E. (2004). *Evaluation: A systematic approach* (7th ed.). Thousand Oaks, CA: Sage.

Sartorius, R., Anderson, T., Bamberger, M., de Garcia, D., Pucilowski, M., & Duthie, M. (2013). *Evaluation: Some tools, methods & approaches*. Retrieved November 16, 2015 from http://www.socialimpact.com/press-releases/DOS-booklet-070213.pdf.

Squires, J., Bricker, D., & Twombly, E. (2002). *Ages & stages questionnaires: Social-emotional*. Baltimore, MD: Paul H. Brooks.

Tebes, J. K., Kaufman, J. S., & Connell, C. M. (2003). The evaluation of prevention and health promotion programs. In T. P. Gullota & M. Bloom (Eds.), *Encyclopedia of primary prevention and health promotion* (pp. 42–61). New York, NY: Springer Science + Business Media.

Chapter 11
Integrating Early Childhood Behavioral Health into Primary Care: The Pediatrician's Perspective

Diane Bloomfield, Nicole Brown, and Karen Warman

Abstract Primary care pediatricians build longitudinal partnerships with families starting in the newborn period, which provide them with opportunities to identify infants and young children at risk for behavioral and developmental disorders and to promote healthy social and emotional development. The American Academy of Pediatrics encourages collaboration between pediatricians and mental health providers to improve pediatric practice by integrating behavioral health providers into the culture of primary care. The required elements include educating pediatric providers about aspects of child social-emotional development, creating workflows to optimize developmental surveillance and screening, and fostering linkages with community-based resources. Through the lens of the primary care pediatrician, we present our experiences integrating the co-located Healthy Steps Program into two large, urban primary care practices in the Bronx, NY. We highlight challenges confronted and successes achieved as we transformed our practices in partnership with our Healthy Steps colleagues.

Keywords Pediatrician • Primary care • American Academy of Pediatrics

Improving Pediatric Practice Through Integrating Behavioral Health for Infants and Young Children

Pediatric primary care clinicians are uniquely suited to identify infants and young children at risk for developmental and behavioral disorders and promote healthy social and emotional development (Committee on Psychosocial Aspects of Child and Family Health and Task Force on Mental Health, 2009). In addition to building longitudinal, trusting, and empowering relationships with families starting in the

D. Bloomfield, M.D. • N. Brown, M.D., M.P.H. (✉) • K. Warman, M.D., M.Sc.
Division of Academic General Pediatrics, Children's Hospital at Montefiore,
Albert Einstein College of Medicine, Bronx, NY, USA
e-mail: dbloomfi@montefiore.org; nicolebr@montefiore.org; kwarman@montefiore.org

© Springer International Publishing Switzerland 2016   181
R.D. Briggs (ed.), *Integrated Early Childhood Behavioral Health in Primary Care*, DOI 10.1007/978-3-319-31815-8_11

newborn period, pediatricians take a developmental approach to health, emphasize preventive care, and are aware of the critical importance of advocacy to promote changes in systems that influence child health and development (Garner, Shonkoff, Committee on Psychosocial Aspects of Child and Family Health, Committee on Early Childhood, Adoption, and Dependent Care, & Section on Developmental and Behavioral Pediatrics, 2012). Pediatricians also understand that a secure and responsive relationship between an infant or toddler and his/her primary caregivers provides a foundation upon which social and emotional development can flourish (Garner et al., 2012). It is now well established that exposure to adverse childhood experiences (ACEs) places a child at high risk for the development of toxic levels of stress that impair neurodevelopment and can lead to chronic, persistent physical and mental health conditions as a child grows into adulthood (Shonkoff, Garner, Committee on Psychosocial Aspects of Child and Family Health, Committee on Early Childhood, Adoption, and Dependent Care, & Section on Developmental and Behavioral Pediatrics, 2012). The American Academy of Pediatrics (AAP) Task Force on Mental Health encourages practice transformation in order to ensure early identification and treatment of developmental and mental health concerns in the medical home (Committee on Psychosocial Aspects of Child and Family Health and Task Force on Mental Health, 2009). In order to expand and improve the provision of mental health services for children, the AAP encourages collaborations between pediatricians and mental health providers to conduct routine developmental and behavioral health screening (Council on Children with Disabilities, Section on Developmental Behavioral Pediatrics, Bright Futures Steering Committee, & Medical Home for Children with Special Needs Project Advisory Committee, 2006), build mental health competencies among primary care clinicians, and foster linkages with community-based resources and services for children with identified concerns and/or for families experiencing significant adversity (Committee on Psychosocial Aspects of Child and Family Health and Task Force on Mental Health, 2009; Garner et al., 2012).

How Will Partnerships Between Pediatricians and Mental Health Providers, Increased Use of Screening Tools, and Increasing Developmental-Behavioral Health Competencies Work in Practice? Examples of Common Concerns Shared by Pediatricians

Many pediatricians working in a busy practice may understandably wonder, "How am I able to take on the additional responsibility of partnering with mental health workers, administering and interpreting screening tools to assess social–emotional development, manage my limited time during office visits to address identified issues, and develop the knowledge and expertise needed to appropriately address mental health concerns?"

When the Healthy Steps Program was first introduced to our practice, there were concerns among the physicians around whether the new Healthy Steps Specialist (HSS) would interfere with our roles as pediatricians. Would the pediatrician become less important? Less autonomous? Was this going to make the visits longer? In addition, many pediatricians were not familiar with some of the screening tools used, such as the Ages and Stages Questionnaires: Social-Emotional (ASQ:SE) (Squires, Bricker, & Twombly, 2002), and had concerns about how universal behavioral/developmental screening would impact our workflow and visits. How would we get parents to fill them out? Did parents have sufficient literacy to do so? How would we become more comfortable with the screening tools and learn more about effectively motivating parents to change their parenting strategy? Would we feel more comfortable with dispensing advice, and what was the current evidence base supporting the advice we gave? We also considered the demands of our schedules, and wondered who would keep track of all of the screenings, administer the age-appropriate screening tool, and score them? Would we have time to counsel families once behavioral health concerns were raised, given our other responsibilities to address a child's physical health, nutrition, growth, immunization status, and other health needs? Would involving the HSS lengthen the time of our visits, keep patients in our waiting or examination rooms longer, and slow our capacity to see patients?

We recognized that in order to effectively integrate early childhood behavioral health into our primary care practices we would need to transform how we delivered care by using a team-based approach. We proposed an approach that provided educational opportunities to pediatricians to increase their familiarity with common developmental and behavioral disorders and assessment and management strategies, implemented universal behavioral/developmental screening among children ages birth to five in our practices, and created workflows that would support integration of these changes into routine pediatric primary care. In order to accomplish this, we met with secretarial, nursing, and clinical staff and designated select staff as champions, developed effective lines of communication, created workflows for universal screening and referrals, and offered educational opportunities to enhance primary care clinicians and staff knowledge about social–emotional development in infants and young children. These changes took place as a result of a collaborative effort between pediatricians, HSS, nurses, and support staff.

Building Competencies in Early Childhood Behavioral Health and Fostering Learning Through Collaborative Care

Studies demonstrate that there is wide variability in the scope and intensity of behavioral health education that pediatric primary care providers (PCPs) receive during their formal training, and that many report low levels of confidence in detecting and managing mental health problems in children younger than 6 years of age (Leaf et al., 2004). In our practices, we sought to build competencies in early childhood behavioral and developmental surveillance and screening by protecting time for pediatricians to learn from HSS about evidence-based tools to screen for and identify common behavioral and developmental disorders in early childhood. Both the AAP and Healthy Steps have developed comprehensive toolkits designed to enhance pediatrician and pediatric resident knowledge about healthy social-emotional development in infancy and early childhood as well as maladaptive development and behaviors (http://healthysteps.zerotothree.org/for-medical-practices-and-other-organizations/healthy-steps-operating-support-materials/. Accessed May 3, 2015; https://www.aap.org/en-us/advocacy-and-policy/aap-health-initiatives/Mental-Health/Pages/Primary-Care-Tools.aspx. Accessed May 3, 2015).

We designed a series of didactic sessions and conferences focused on screening tools that measure child (birth to 5) social-emotional development, such as the ASQ:SE (Squires et al., 2002) and the Modified Checklist for Autism in Toddlers-Revised (MCHAT-R) (Robins et al., 2014). These didactic sessions were often facilitated by a HSS, developmental pediatrician, or other pediatric provider with specific expertise in infant and early childhood development. We also addressed topics such as assessing "joint attention" in the evaluation of autism, "the power of attention" in behavioral management, common behavioral concerns such as managing tantrums, and the impact of ACEs on parenting and child development. Our Healthy Steps colleagues delivered many of these lectures to medical students, interns, and residents.

Regular, bidirectional communication between pediatricians and the Healthy Steps team is critical to foster a culture of collaborative care, and ensure appropriate referrals to community supports and services for infants and young children with identified concerns (Chenven, 2010). Direct consultation during pediatric visits from an infant and child development expert enhances provider capacity to assess and manage developmental and social-emotional disorders (Briggs et al., 2012). Consultations can take place jointly with the family, PCP, and HSS, or the HSS can meet with the family before the visit with their pediatrician. The pediatricians in our practices found that the HSS could model for us approaches to certain problems. They often discussed with us which approach to a behavioral concern they took, and why. For example, the HSS will often meet with the family before the pediatrician sees them, and have identified a concern, such as sleeping, and will have already started to discuss strategies with the family. This promotes family-centered care, as parents feel that their concerns have been heard and are being addressed. It also relieves the pediatrician of having to discuss sleep in greater depth, as he or she knows that the family already received appropriate guidance. The HSS often provides a summary of the conversation for the physician so that he or she can also reinforce this guidance with the family and support the plan to change sleep hygiene. Notes documented by HSS were easily accessible to us in our electronic medical record system, which further enhanced our understanding of the approach taken and guidance given to a family. In addition, we could ask the family to reflect back to us the advice they had been given during a visit with the Healthy Steps professional.

To ensure bidirectional communication, the pediatricians in our practice commonly share their insights and approaches to the biopsychosocial needs of the family with the integrated behavioral health team members. HSS will then often discuss therapeutic strategies they will implement with a family, as well as community resources and supports that may be appropriate for the family. This allows the team to participate in problem-based learning, including observing how a problem presents, understanding how a management approach is presented to a family, and learning more details about the parents' own ACEs or ongoing challenges. Pediatricians in our practice can read HSS notes and help facilitate scheduling follow-up visits with the family to evaluate progress and outcomes. Readily available consultants and joint clinical visits have helped our practices optimize learning, information sharing, and a culture of collaboration.

The proximity of team members is an important element of an effective integration plan. It is essential that the medical and integrated behavioral health team be physically co-located. This arrangement enhances a warm handoff where the pediatrician can introduce the family to the behavioral health team member and outline the ways the two providers will be working together. A number of studies have substantiated that the "warm handoff" reduces stigma associated with mental healthcare, and significantly improves patient engagement in care (Horevitz, Organista, & Arean, 2015). The physical proximity encourages curbside consultations between providers and the behavioral health provider. This increasing familiarity and easy accessibility is key to building a trusting, respectful, and successful collaboration.

Designing Screening and Patient Care Workflows That Foster Integration of Behavioral Health Providers in Pediatric Primary Care

The initial meeting with key staff members should occur before the creation of any workflows. This is an opportunity to select champions in each of the domains who will facilitate the integration of the new team members. These champions from the secretarial, nursing, and physician cadre can share important insights with the behavioral health team about the best strategies to increase the buy-in of their fellow staff towards the successful implementation of change within the practice. These preliminary meetings will reinforce the important role that all levels of staff will contribute towards identifying individuals who are at risk and could benefit from a behavioral health intervention. Many of the secretarial and nursing team members will note interactions in the waiting area between parents and their children, and it is important that they feel empowered to alert providers to these families. These frontline observations will aid in the overall collaborative nature of care in the practice.

One main barrier to utilizing screening tools and providing care to children with social-emotional difficulties, cited by primary care physicians, is the time constraints of the general well-child visit (King & Glascoe, 2003). Universal screening will require additional time and new responsibilities for all members of the pediatric practice. In order to incorporate universal screening and the behavioral health team into the primary care practice, workflows must be developed that take into account the culture of your individual practice. To become truly integrated into a team, all members must be aware/accepting of the positive opportunities that this collaboration can bring to their daily interactions with the patients they serve.

As described, an important first step in the workflow for addressing the behavioral health needs of the infant and child is the universal screening of this population to determine which families might benefit from the team's services. In a busy practice, screening can be accomplished if the stakeholders are committed to incorporating these tools into their daily practice. In some cases, the champions can advocate for this process after completing the tools using their own experiences as parents. They may then have additional insight into the definition of best practices for their sites, and may more successfully emphasize the benefits of screening tools for the patient population.

A successful workflow can utilize the electronic medical record as a prompt to remind the staff about which screening tools are to be used at each visit. The front desk staff and nursing personnel can help reduce the amount of time spent on the screens by ensuring that the parents complete the screening surveys in the waiting or exam rooms while they are waiting to be seen by the physician. In our practices, this began during registration, where front desk staff learned to be mindful of the patient's age and give the parents the appropriate screening tool for the child. The nursing staff can input the data into the electronic medical record, which allows the provider to quickly identify any areas of particular concern. These screening tools and associated workflows help our providers to identify issues in a systematic way that might otherwise have been missed during routine care. Pediatricians could then initiate a referral or get direct consultation from the HSS based on the result of a positive screen or other concern elicited during this process. The use of screening tools also sets the tone for the visit, as families understand that we are interested in the child's social and emotional skills in addition to their other medical concerns.

The champions or first-adopters are able to feedback to the entire team the ways that effective screening can save time for the practice and improve patient satisfaction. Early identification of developmental disabilities has been proven to improve the long-term outcome of children and their families, yet in a recent study, only 61 % of patients who had abnormal screens were referred for care (King et al., 2010). An integrated system that provides prompt assessment and treatment of challenging cases by a skilled behavioral health expert, can reduce time spent by primary care clinicians searching for a referral source for these patients.

All integrated systems should have clinical information systems that support proactive planning and informed decision-making. Electronic health records help to facilitate data collection, and enable a practice to perform surveillance around quality metrics such as rates of developmental screening and referrals to clinic and community-based patient and family supports and services among a population of patients. An integrated clinic may consider measuring other patient and family-level outcomes, including parent mental and child developmental/social-emotional outcomes, to ensure that evidence-based interventions are efficacious and effective. Patient and provider satisfaction surveys also help to facilitate practice improvement and should be an important part of quality initiatives. Finally, pediatric providers can utilize and refine the multidisciplinary care plan to ensure that services continue to be tailored appropriately and delivered effectively.

At our site, we tracked the timely completion of ASQs and other screening tools in order to track our success in implementation. If surveys were not being completed, we worked with the staff to troubleshoot obstacles to successful completion. If we were doing well, we gave recognition to the staff for a job well done to encourage ongoing compliance. Our patient satisfaction surveys confirmed that the parents felt respected and heard by the Healthy Steps team and valued the program.

Benefits of Integrating Early Childhood Behavioral Health into Pediatric Primary Care: The Montefiore Experience

Increased attention to infant and early childhood behavioral–developmental health has led to expected increases in detection and referrals for developmental and behavioral concerns as well as increased parenting support, attention to parent mental health and focus on parenting skills development. Parents feel supported and are appreciative of the care given. Members of the team who help in implementing the program take pride in the work that they are doing. Primary care clinicians have gained increased comfort and skill in detecting and addressing developmental, behavioral, and mental health concerns. In addition to the direct effects of early detection and referral for developmental–behavioral health concerns, we found that continuity of care increased, we forged stronger relationships with community-based resources including mental health services for parents and early intervention providers, and we increased our provision of family-centered care.

Increasing Continuity of Care

Partnering with the integrated behavioral health team allows for the provision of longitudinal multidisciplinary care that continues after the office visit. The behavioral health provider may follow up with the family by phone or make referrals to community-based services. In our clinic, having the HSS serve as a physician extender relieves the pediatrician of some of the follow-up work required to coordinate care and services, or assess outcomes outside of an office visit. The HSS also acts a bridge for families to their pediatricians or other mental health specialists and service providers involved in the care of the child. A mother might not know how to reach her child's pediatrician quickly for help with a concern. The HSS is often readily available, and can help to triage a parent's concern, and communicate that concern quickly to the child's pediatrician. In addition, because the Healthy Steps provider encourages the patient and family to follow up with their primary care doctor, continuity of care is supported. Families who might normally end up seeing several different doctors, and not identifying a particular physician as their child's doctor, are more likely to have a sustained relationship with a particular physician.

Enhancing Community Resources and Referrals for Socially Complex Families

Integrated early childhood behavioral health providers have a wealth of knowledge with respect to early intervention programs and community resources for infants and children with developmental disorders or social-emotional concerns. Potential community linkages can be shared during didactic conferences, in a resource guide within the clinic, or during patient consultations.

For families with multiple psychosocial stressors, and those who have infants with complex medical and developmental needs, a multidisciplinary care team with the capacity to coordinate care and services is an essential component of delivering integrated care. In our pediatric practice, this team generally consists of a PCP, the HSS, and a social worker. If an infant or child screens positive for a possible developmental delay, presents with a behavioral concern, or is exposed to multiple psychosocial stressors that may impair their development and overall social-emotional health, the PCP should have ready access to these team members, who in turn help facilitate linkages to community-based services and supports such as mental health counseling for parents, early intervention, behavioral therapy, and supports to optimize housing and food security.

Family-Centered Care

A family-centered, comprehensive patient/family care plan is an important outcome of the Healthy Steps program—that is, the family is fully engaged in defining goals of care and the type of services to be delivered. In addition, the mode of clinical communication between the practice team and the behavioral health team must be designed to facilitate bidirectional feedback about their shared patients. This is another example of the advantage of an electronic medical record as a useful way for the pediatricians to send queries about their patients and review the assessment and plan created by the behavioral health team. The care plan is often shared with team members and other subspecialty providers in the patient's electronic medical record, thereby optimizing the ability to communicate and coordinate patient care.

Summary

Pediatricians in our practices have embraced HSS, our behavioral health colleagues, as our partners, not our replacements. We have seen that a team-based approach to surveillance, screening, and management of developmental and behavioral disorders in early childhood has greatly improved screening rates and timely referrals to early intervention and other critical services. In addition to improving services and care for our patients, we have come to appreciate the time and expertise required to understand why parents have adopted their current parenting techniques and have learned to encourage parents to adopt more positive and less punitive parenting strategies. While some parents may benefit from basic support with parenting skills, others have far greater needs. Over the past 10 years since we have had HSS integrated into our practice, we have successfully worked together to support parents with a variety of challenges, including severe mental illness, their own history of abuse, lack of social support, literacy issues, and cognitive impairment. These parents, who previously would have been unlikely to establish consistent, ongoing relationships with a particular pediatrician, are now more likely to come in regularly for routine visits because they have an additional consistent advisor and source of support on the care team.

We have found that by creating a culture of mutual respect, enhancing provider and staff education and working together to create practice workflows, we could collaborate together in ways that respect our time, take advantage of our different skill sets, and deliver innumerable benefits to our families. Our practice has transformed to fully integrate parenting skills and behavioral health supports into the routine care that we provide, and as pediatricians, we take pride in knowing that we offer comprehensive care and supports designed to optimize the social and emotional growth of the infants and young children we care for.

References

Briggs, R. D., Stettler, E. M., Silver, E. J., Schrag, R. D., Nayak, M., Chinitz, S., & Racine, A. D. (2012). Social emotional screening for infants and toddlers in primary care. *Pediatrics, 129*(2), e377–e384.

Chenven, M. (2010). Community systems of care for children's mental health. *Child and Adolescent Psychiatric Clinics of North America, 19*(1), 163–174.

Committee on Psychosocial Aspects of Child and Family Health and Task Force on Mental Health. (2009). Policy statement—The future of pediatrics: Mental health competencies for pediatric primary care. *Pediatrics, 124*(1), 410–421.

Council on Children with Disabilities, Section on Developmental Behavioral Pediatrics, Bright Futures Steering Committee, & Medical Home for Children with Special Needs Project Advisory Committee. (2006). Identifying infants and young children with developmental disorders in the medical home: An algorithm for developmental surveillance and screening. *Pediatrics, 118*(1), 405–420.

Garner, A. S., Shonkoff, J. P., Committee on Psychosocial Aspects of Child and Family Health, Committee on Early Childhood, Adoption, and Dependent Care, & Section on Developmental and Behavioral Pediatrics. (2012). Early childhood adversity, toxic stress, and the role of the pediatrician: Translating developmental science into lifelong health. *Pediatrics, 129*(1), e224–e231.

Horevitz, E., Organista, K. C., & Arean, P. A. (2015). Depression treatment uptake in integrated primary care: How a warm handoff and other factors affect decision making by Latinos. *Psychiatric Services, 66*(4), 824–830. doi:10.1176/appi.ps.201400085.

King, T. M., & Glascoe, F. P. (2003). Developmental surveillance of infants and young children in pediatric primary care. *Current Opinion in Pediatrics, 15*(6), 624–629.

King, T. M., Tandon, S. D., Macias, M. M., Healy, J. A., Duncan, P. M., Swigonski, N. L., ... Lipkin, P. H. (2010). Implementing developmental screening and referrals: Lessons learned from a national project. *Pediatrics, 125*(2), 350–360.

Leaf, P. J., Owens, P. M., Leventhal, J. M., Forsyth, B. W., Vaden-Kiernan, M., Epstein, L. D., …
    Horwitz, S. M. (2004). Pediatricians' training and identification and management of psychoso-
    cial problems. *Clinical Pediatrics, 43*(4), 355–365.
Robins, D. L., Casagrande, K., Barton, M., Chen, C. M., Dumont-Matheiu, T., & Fein, D. (2014).
    Validation of the modified checklist for Autism in toddler, revised with follow-up (M-CHAT-
    R/F). *Pediatrics, 133*(1), 37–45.
Shonkoff, J. P., Garner, A. S., Committee on Psychosocial Aspects of Child and Family Health,
    Committee on Early Childhood, Adoption, and Dependent Care, & Section on Developmental
    and Behavioral Pediatrics. (2012). The lifelong effects of early childhood adversity and toxic
    stress. *Pediatrics, 129*(1), e232–e246.
Squires, J., Bricker, D., & Twombly, E. (2002). *The ASQ:SE user's guide for the ages & stages
    questionnaires®: Social-emotional: A parent-completed, child-monitoring system for social-
    emotional behaviors*. Baltimore, MD: Paul H. Brookes.

Chapter 12
Stories from the Exam Room: Case Examples of Healthy Steps Interventions at Montefiore

Laura Krug and Polina Umylny

Abstract Healthy Steps at Montefiore follows the integrated care model in which clinically trained behavioral health professionals, with expertise in early childhood development, trauma, and attachment theory, are embedded within general pediatrics practices to meet with families in a universally accessed, non-stigmatized setting. Healthy Steps Specialists intervene at three levels to address the multiple concerns that families bring to their child's pediatrician. First, Healthy Steps Specialists implement a universal screening program, working alongside pediatricians to identify families of infants with historical or current psychosocial stressors, and provide services intended to prevent the transmission of trauma across generations. Healthy Steps Specialists also work with families of children, aged birth to 5, who require short-term interventions related to concerns about behavior and development, including difficulties with feeding, sleep, tantrums, and aggression. Finally, Healthy Steps Specialists provide mental health interventions to parents of very young children in order to address concerns that may impede a parent's ability to attend to their children's developmental needs. Four vignettes included in this chapter offer examples of these levels of intervention.

Keywords Healthy Steps • Integrated behavioral health • Early childhood • ACEs • Maternal trauma

Healthy Steps at Montefiore follows the integrated care model in which clinically trained behavioral health professionals, with expertise in early childhood development, trauma, and attachment theory, are embedded within general pediatrics practices to meet with families in a universally accessed, non-stigmatized setting.

Healthy Steps Specialists intervene at three levels to address the multiple concerns that families bring to their child's pediatrician:

L. Krug, L.C.S.W. (✉) • P. Umylny, Ph.D. (✉)
Montefiore Health System, Bronx, NY, USA
e-mail: lkrug@montefiore.org; pumylny@montefiore.org

© Springer International Publishing Switzerland 2016
R.D. Briggs (ed.), *Integrated Early Childhood Behavioral Health in Primary Care*, DOI 10.1007/978-3-319-31815-8_12

1. Healthy Steps Intensive Services: Healthy Steps Specialists, working alongside pediatricians, implement a universal screening program, to identify families of infants with historical or current psychosocial stressors, and provide services intended to prevent the transmission of trauma across generations. Families can also be identified prenatally when mothers attend their obstetric appointments.
2. Healthy Steps Consultations: Healthy Steps Specialists work with families of children, aged birth to 5, who require short-term interventions (approximately one to five sessions) related to concerns about behavior and development. Children can be referred for a variety of reasons including difficulties with feeding, sleep, tantrums, and aggression.
3. Parental Mental Health: Healthy Steps Specialists provide mental health interventions to parents of very young children in order to address concerns that may impede a parent's ability to attend to their children's developmental needs. Parental Mental Health Providers provide evidence-based individual therapy to the parent, while always keeping the parent–child dyad in mind.

The four vignettes included in this chapter are examples of these levels of intervention. All names have been changed to protect confidentiality.

Intensive Services

Intensive Services works particularly well when babies are referred very early, sometimes even prenatally, and Healthy Steps Specialists are able to meet families at the newborn visit or soon after, when parents are overwhelmed, exhausted, and deeply humbled by the birth of their baby. The following vignette is based on a family enrolled in Healthy Steps Intensive Services at a Montefiore pediatric clinic in the Bronx, NY.

After completing the well-baby checkup on 1-month-old Genie, Dr. Johnson came to find the Healthy Steps Specialist.[1] Genie was the youngest of four girls being raised by Luisa, a single mother. Dr. Johnson had been caring for Genie's three older sisters for several years, and knew that Luisa and her children had spent the last 9 years moving between homeless shelters in three of New York City's five boroughs. In addition, Genie had been born early and underweight, had spent several weeks in the NICU, and Luisa was clearly anxious about her infant's well-being. Dr. Johnson appropriately thought the family could benefit from the support of the Intensive Services program and made the referral.

After the "warm handoff" with Dr. Johnson, Luisa agreed to meet with me in the exam room. As many parents do, Luisa had a great deal of trust in her children's pediatrician, and was willing to accept her endorsement of me as a respected

---

[1] Adapted from "Integrating Behavioral Health Support Into a Pediatric Setting: What Happens in the Exam Room?," K. Cuno, L. M. Krug, and P. Umylny, 2015, *Zero to Three, 35*(6) p. 11–16. Copyright 2015 by ZERO TO THREE. Adapted with permission.

colleague. The primary goals at this first meeting are to establish rapport with the parent and to provide concrete examples of how enrollment in Intensive Services would be helpful for the family. It is also an opportunity to observe the parent–child relationship at a very early point in its development.

I explained that I was a Healthy Steps Specialist, available to answer additional questions, review typical newborn milestones, and introduce Luisa to fundamental concepts regarding brain development. I also mentioned that I hoped to ask Luisa questions about her childhood experiences. Luisa was open to meeting with me and I began by asking how she was doing and if she had any questions or concerns about caring for Genie. From our first meeting it was evident how anxious Luisa was about Genie's health. We discussed these worries so that Luisa would know that this was an appropriate context in which to address such concerns, and I worked to ensure that Luisa felt heard. I provided information on strategies for feeding and soothing Genie and Luisa was able to practice these techniques in the exam room during our session. There was no time to explore Luisa's history during this first meeting, but fortunately integration into pediatrics almost always ensures that families will return soon, due to the well-child visit schedule.

Luisa and Genie returned to the clinic the following week for a weight check, and Luisa was thrilled to report that Genie seemed to be eating more and had put on some weight. I encouraged her to notice how Genie's behavior had changed since birth. She noted, with some regret, that Genie frequently seemed angry, only smiling in her sleep or when looking up at the light. I noticed mother's negative attribution as potentially indicative of relationships from her past, and we discussed how a baby's smile was reflexive at this age and that over the next few weeks it would develop into a social smile. Luisa appeared relieved and I inquired if she had been warned by friends or family to be careful not to spoil Genie. Luisa agreed and stated, "I even tell the girls to put the baby down, but they don't always listen." Luisa also confessed, "I can't help it, she's just so small. I know I should let her cry it out but I can't stand it." This was the perfect opportunity to debunk the prevalent myth that soothing young babies creates excessive dependence, and support Luisa's innate need to respond to her baby's cues to nurture Genie.

I discussed the "serve and return" nature of brain development, how Genie learned from the responses she consistently received from her caregivers, and that when Luisa soothed Genie over and over again, Genie would gradually learn to sooth herself. My goal during these discussions was to support the development of a secure attachment between parents and babies by encouraging Luisa to imagine how the security Genie felt from Luisa as a baby would serve Genie well as she grew older. Providing an accessible explanation of brain science and explaining that brain development in infancy was the foundation for all later learning is a crucial component of early Healthy Steps visits. I encouraged Luisa to reflect on Genie's current capabilities and acknowledge how completely dependent she was, and that Luisa was not creating a dependency, but appropriately meeting Genie's needs. Finally, I explained the difference between nurturing a young baby versus "indulging" a toddler and explained how a consistently nurtured baby develops into a more independent child.

Luisa seemed eager to hear this. "It's okay to hold the baby?" she asked to confirm. "Absolutely! Not only is it okay to hold the baby, it's great to hold the baby." Luisa's relief was palpable. "We can work together, when you come in to see Dr. Johnson, to see how things are going, and to discuss how you care for Genie. Over time, I will encourage you to gradually allow Genie to tolerate some frustration. But for now, nurture her as much as you can." I stressed that she would decide exactly how to raise her baby and her children. I explained that I would offer information, and support her and her family, regardless of her decisions.

At this visit, I also had the opportunity to complete the Adverse Childhood Experiences (ACEs) questionnaire (Felitti et al., 1998). When Healthy Steps Specialists first began screening parents with the ACEs, we were apprehensive about asking personal and often painful information about their pasts. While not all parents reveal a history of childhood trauma, many do. I introduced the screening to Luisa by noting that many parents at our clinic had a "rough go" as kids, and that research tells us trauma tends to repeat generation after generation. I explained that our goal was to support parents who experienced trauma as kids, in an effort to prevent repetition in this generation, our patients. "It's true," Luisa said. "There is a lot of that in my family." I began by asking Luisa who raised her and she reported being cared for by multiple family members until she moved out on her own at age 16. She endorsed both physical and emotional abuse and noted that her single mother was largely absent and addicted to drugs. Luisa described her story in a minimalist and matter of fact manner, as if she did not want to give the memory too much credence. She explained that she preferred not think about her past, and she was clearly more focused on her children's well-being than her own. She denied any history of her own drug abuse, mental illness, or domestic violence.

The ACEs screening is not a comprehensive psychosocial history, but we believe that it is useful to identify parents at high risk for challenges with attachment and repetition of abuse. In addition to identifying those babies most at risk, screening can bring the painful and often deeply hidden memories into the present, where they can be openly addressed. I have never met a parent who thought their baby was at risk for abuse, and the parents who can speak about their abuse histories with their Healthy Steps Specialist may be the most resilient in preventing its repetition. The families who refuse to answer the questions, or fail to acknowledge the trauma they experienced, may be the most vulnerable. However, there is always another opportunity to connect them with Healthy Steps at their next visit to the pediatrician when their doctor may observe a small comment or gesture suggesting the vulnerabilities that lie beneath the surface.

I met with Genie and Luisa a few weeks later at the 2-month checkup. Luisa happily reported that Genie was continuing to gain weight and was smiling socially, cooing, and kicking enthusiastically when Luisa or the other girls played with her. Despite these developmental milestones, Genie's health was an ongoing struggle during her first year of life, with several hospitalizations and frequent trips to the emergency room. When Genie came for her many pediatric appointments, Luisa and I met to see how she and the girls were managing. In the absence of a family crisis, Luisa spoke almost exclusively about Genie. Though Luisa was devoted to her three older daughters, I doubted that they were able to see this devotion past Luisa's sleep deprivation and irritability.

In my work with parents, I spend much of my time encouraging them to interpret and respond to their infant's language, much like I did in the first few sessions with Luisa. As the months went on, however, I veered in a slightly different direction, encouraging Luisa to identify times when she could, quite literally, look up from her singular focus on Genie, so that she could better address the needs of her older children. She was not convinced when, at the 6-month visit, I suggested that giving Genie a chance to problem solve, soothe, or entertain herself was important for her development, but she agreed to implement the strategies I recommended and "see what happens."

While Luisa doted on Genie, she expected her older daughters to embrace her own approach to life: live up to your responsibilities and count your blessings. This philosophy left little room for limit testing or even playfulness. It was only a matter of time before Luisa's anxiety over Genie's health would shift to frustration over her burgeoning independence. Consequently, we spoke a great deal about limit setting in very young children. At the 9-month well-child visit, when Luisa began to describe Genie as "demanding…just like her older sister," referring to 4-year-old Leah, I acknowledged that caring for the needs of very young children can be depleting, and we spoke about how her children's strong mindedness can also serve them well in life. I pointed out that I saw the same streak of independence and perseverance in Luisa, and how those attributes had helped her overcome many of life's obstacles. At this same visit we learned that the family had been moved to a shelter in Brooklyn, though Luisa was continuing to take the subway and several busses to get the older girls to their schools in the Bronx, and continued to bring her family to our clinic for their medical care. Between pediatric and Healthy Steps visits, Dr. Johnson and I wrote letters and made phone calls to the Department of Homeless Services, requesting that the family get a medical transfer to a shelter closer to the clinic, so that Genie could continue to receive medical care at her established medical home.

By the 12-month visit, the family had been moved back to the Bronx, but the toll of life between boroughs had worn away at the family's ability to cope. When we met after Genie's physical, Luisa told me that 14-year-old Carlie was cutting school and "having sex with boys" in stairwells of buildings. In the midst of the family's daily struggles, Carlie had been given more responsibility for caring for her younger siblings than she was ready for, and she directed her anger at Luisa. Luisa shared how much she feared for Carlie's future. With her own history of abuse and trauma, Luisa had struggled to create a different life for her daughters. Carlie's behavior was, for Luisa, evidence that she had failed, and that all four of her children were destined to repeat her own life course. I worked with Luisa to remind her of the ways in which she had already made her daughters' lives different from her own childhood experiences. She had avoided abusive relationships, limited her children's exposure to violence and drug use, and kept their days as routine and consistent as possible, within the limitations of life in the shelter. I encouraged Luisa to accept a referral for therapy, both for Carlie and herself, but she insisted that she would be able to manage the difficulties on her own.

When I walked in to the exam room to meet with the family 6 months later, at Genie's 18-month-old well-child visit, I found Genie sitting on the exam table, with Luisa standing by protectively. Carlie and Leah were attempting to read Genie a story, while Genie seemed intent on claiming the book as her own. I also learned that the family had some good news to share. Carlie bubbled over with enthusiasm to tell me that the family had finally moved out of the shelter and into their own apartment. As we celebrated the family's new home, Luisa followed this news with another accomplishment. "Carlie is on the honor roll!" Luisa told me, with more relief than pride. This news, and Luisa's enthusiasm in sharing it with me, seemed like a good barometer of how well the family was doing.

During this visit, I also noted that Luisa had started to describe Genie as "smart and independent," and had begun to allow Genie to do more on her own. She also spoke more kindly and less harshly to her older children. I pointed out that Luisa was doing an admirable job letting the girls work out the conflict over the book, and that her daughters were showing strong negotiation skills. When I revisited concerns about limit setting, Leah chimed in, "She keeps hitting me!" I agreed that 18-month-olds can be impatient and easily frustrated, and pointed out that Genie may not yet have the words to express herself fully and so may lash out instead. We spoke about the power of attention, both parental and sibling, to shape behavior, and to teach Genie to start to identify and express her feelings. I also stressed the importance of immediate and logical consequences, and the older girls "practiced" how they would respond to Genie the next time she hit.

The visit ended as positively for the family as it began, and I stressed that Luisa and her children had all worked hard to get to this point, with so many successes to share. We reviewed upcoming milestones, and Luisa and I agreed to meet at Genie's next checkup.

While Genie's family presented well in the snapshot of this visit, I knew that they had many hurdles ahead. Working in an integrated pediatric setting, Healthy Steps Specialists have the luxury of knowing that we will see families on a regular basis, as attendance at pediatric appointments is a priority for most parents. In addition, because families remain enrolled in our program until the child's fifth birthday, Healthy Steps Specialists are able to work with families over an extended period, allowing opportunities for families to make significant changes during a child's most vulnerable phase of development.

This aspect of the program became critical 1 month after Genie's 18-month visit. Luisa had discovered that Carlie had continued to have sex with multiple partners, and brought her in to the clinic for pregnancy and STD tests. While Carlie met with her pediatrician, Luisa, Genie, and I met in my office. Importantly, at this visit, both Luisa and Carlie agreed to a referral for therapy. Because of our integrated model, I was able to introduce Luisa and Carlie to the clinic's pediatric social worker, who was able to schedule an appointment for the following week. When Luisa brought Carlie in for that appointment, she also agreed to meet with Dr. Bassett, our Parental Mental Health Psychologist. While Luisa was always eager to implement any strategies that I suggested, overwhelmed by her traumatic history and chaotic circumstances, she often struggled to understand things from her children's perspective. I hoped that becoming involved in her own treatment would enable her to be more empathic towards her children.

Behavior and Development Consultation

Healthy Steps consultations integrated in general pediatrics benefit both families and pediatricians. Parents frequently seek help from pediatricians, asking advice on a myriad of behavioral and developmental issues. Pediatricians, in turn, often feel as if they have neither the time nor the expertise to address these concerns effectively. Providing behavioral health and developmental specialists allows for a more holistic approach to pediatric care, allowing providers to identify and treat children's difficulties early, before those difficulties become both exacerbated and entrenched.

Ms. Castillo brought her 3-year-old son, Michael, to see the pediatrician when his daycare center threatened to kick him out due to poor behavior and aggression. She and her husband were raising Michael and her three boys (ages 4, 7, and 12 years old) from a previous relationship. Dr. Edwards referred the family to Healthy Steps, and due to time constraints, after a brief introduction, we scheduled a consultation for the following week. I noticed that the family had been referred the year before, with the same concerns, but the parents never followed through with their first appointment. I imagined that Michael's behaviors at 2, without the benefit of intervention, had become very challenging.

Michael entered my office with a bright and friendly smile. He immediately began to play with toys, talking happily and showing his parents his discoveries. Mr. and Mrs. Castillo redirected Michael from time to time to return toys before taking out new ones. Michael was compliant with their requests and demonstrated no defiance during our discussion. Michael's parents reported that their home was very busy with four boys, but that Michael was the only one who gave them much trouble. They reported that they had a daily routine including homework time, bath time, dinner, and free play. I was impressed with the significant structure they had created. They noted that they both worked full time and that Michael's maternal grandmother watched the older boys until Mrs. Castillo came home in the evening, picking up Michael from daycare on her way.

The Castillos reported that Michael was always "hyper," ignored their directions, and had explosive tantrums when he did not get his way. Michael's behavior at school was similar, and included bullying and aggression toward the other children. They added that Michael resisted their attempts to create routines, and that bedtime, in particular, had become a series of battles. Michael also often woke up in the middle of the night to play or raid the refrigerator. They voiced concern that Michael was a danger to himself when he was up at night unsupervised. Recently, they woke up one morning to find he had hidden a take-out container under his pillow and had a face covered in bar-b-que sauce. Mr. Castillo noted that he had been diagnosed with ADHD as a child and feared that Michael had it as well. I immediately felt empathy for this dad, who was raising three well-behaved stepchildren, and struggling with his own.

I began my response by establishing ground rules, explaining that Healthy Steps behavior and development consultations at our clinic were limited to a few visits, and that patients who required more interventions were referred out. I ruled out that Michael had been exposed to any trauma in his short life, such as domestic violence, parental mental illness, substance abuse, child abuse or neglect. Screening all consultations for trauma is an important step as posttraumatic stress reactions are frequently misdiagnosed as hyperactivity and defiance. I explained that Michael was too young to be diagnosed with ADHD, and normalized some of Michael's high activity as typical of children his age. I applauded the Castillos for coming to the appointment, as early intervention is critical. I noted that if Michael's behaviors persisted and interfered with his ability to learn once he was in school, they could request a psychoeducational evaluation through the school district.

I explained that multiple factors affect children's behavior, including temperament, developmental stage, their caregiving environment, past experiences, and consequences (both positive and negative) for behavior. I commended the Castillos on their efforts to maintain a calm and structured home, with four young sons, and noted that it appeared that Michael required a different kind of parenting than his siblings.

Next, I worked to get a sense of what strategies the Castillos were already using to manage Michael's behavior, and I clarified how the Castillos attempted to establish limits. Both parents agreed that they did not give any consistent consequence when Michael ignored their efforts to enforce routines and limits. The Castillos did not hit their children, but were at a loss about what to do instead. The Castillos had both been raised with corporal punishment, had made a conscious decision to parent differently, and were frustrated that Michael's behavior seemed to discredit their theory that respectful parenting would be rewarded with well-behaved children.

I noted that while in my office, and without the challenge of competing for attention, Michael seemed to have little difficulty with compliance, and played in a calm and well-organized manner. Mr. Castillo noted that he could not remember the last time when being with Michael was so calm and peaceful. They agreed that during this discussion, Michael had been getting a great deal of support and attention from his parents, and acknowledged that, with two jobs and four children, sitting in a room just with Michael and allowing him to play was its own novelty.

This discussion allowed for an introduction of the importance of parental attention in shaping children's behaviors. We discussed the importance of giving Michael lots of positive attention when he behaved well, and to remove their attention when he misbehaved. The Castillos spoke about how ineffective they felt as parents, and I stressed that Michael, like most children, would continue to show them the behaviors that they pay the most attention to, and that by using a combination of planned ignoring and positive attention, they could start to shift Michael's behaviors.

As an example, we worked to identify two problem behaviors, spoke about what the "positive opposite" of those behaviors might be, and discussed how to use language (in particular, specific praise and narrating Michael's positive behaviors) to reinforce the behaviors that the Castillos were looking for. Armed with these strategies and a few carefully selected handouts, I asked the Castillos to practice these skills in the office, while playing with Michael and following his lead. The Castillos were good sports, and were quickly speaking over each other in an effort to identify Michael's positive behaviors. Although initially reluctant to commit to similar activities at home, explaining that they had so little time to get everything done in a day as it was, both parents agreed that at least one of them would be able to play with Michael in this way every day in order to practice the skills we had discussed today. I stressed that spending a few minutes playing with Michael, and following his lead, would be important. These 5-min "special play time sessions" add up quickly and ensure that parents have time set aside to foster a strong relationship with their child.

We then discussed how they could apply some of the strategies we had discussed today to avoid and manage Michael's tantrums. I stressed how "giving in" to Michael's tantrums, because it was difficult for both of his parents to tolerate his distress, was actually encouraging more tantrums. I suggested that when Michael had tantrums, they explain to him that he would finish his tantrum in his room and come out when done.

Although it had been a full session and we were running short on time, I felt obliged to address their concerns regarding Michael's nighttime adventures, and suggested that attaching a bell or other noise creating object to his bedroom door would wake one of them up and remove the secrecy of his behavior. The Castillos, although actively engaged in the visit, voiced feeling skeptical that any changes they made would have an impact on Michael's out of control behavior. We agreed to meet next week to check their progress and revisit these concerns.

At the next session, the Castillos reported that they had diligently practiced their skills during playtime with Michael. Michael was eager to tell me that he enjoyed the special time with his parents, and his parents agreed that his behavior was very different during these play sessions. They also reported successfully directing Michael to his room during tantrums. Ms. Castillo voiced amazement after noticing how much calmer she felt when the tantrums were not occurring at her feet. While this change gave them hope for more change to come, they were concerned that shifting their attention alone would not address all of Michael's behavioral difficulties. I agreed and explained that in this session we would focus on setting limits and rules, giving effective commands, and following through on consequences, both when Michael complied and when he ignored or defied their limits.

We identified specific rules that the Castillos wanted Michael to follow and they both agreed that his aggressive behavior was their greatest concern. "Keeping hands and feet safe" became a family rule that Michael and his parents could all agree on. I suggested that they immediately put Michael into a time out, well away from any family activity, after aggression. We discussed giving Michael clear and consistent warnings for non-aggressive misbehavior, by giving him three chances, or "strikes," and that if they said the words "strike three" he received a time out. We also discussed setting up a chart of the series of activities around bedtime, so that Michael could check off each step as he completed it.

Throughout this session, I gave very explicit recommendations to the Castillos, checking in with them to make sure that the recommended strategies seemed fair and kind. I encouraged them to continue to track Michael's progress, and to focus on the changes that Michael was making in his behavior, rather than on what they still wanted to change.

At Michael's third visit, he immediately began to play with the toys and the Castillos reported that they were seeing some results. While Michael continued to be extremely demanding and had a hard time sharing, he was staying in his room during tantrums and standing in the hallway for time outs. Mr. Castillo voiced amazement that Michael complied with their directions during time outs.

During our conversation about Michael's improvements, I noticed that he was quietly tossing blocks from the bin over his right shoulder, onto the floor. Mrs. Castillo quickly told him to stop, which he ignored. I reminded mom to clearly define her limits by giving him a first strike warning and encouraged them to discuss where the time out spot would be in my office. Michael ignored the strikes and cried while standing in corner for his time out. I restarted the timer after he kicked a toy and he remained quiet in the corner for the duration of his 3 min. We commended Michael for calming himself down and his father reminded him why he received the time out in the first place, finishing the statement with the question "Are you ready to play nicely with the toys?" Michael nodded and perfectly illustrated his capacity for self-control.

As Michael returned proudly to his activity, we discussed his progress up to this point. Mrs. Castillo confessed that she had not embraced the recommendations as quickly as her husband. She noted that she had a harder time controlling her frustration and tended to send Michael to his room without the three strikes or clearly defined time outs. Mr. Castillo proudly observed that the more control he felt, the more effective his discipline was; "We are talking more and yelling less." Ms. Castillo agreed that Michael was responding so well to the structure and limits, that it was as if he wanted them. I agreed and noted that although young children desire control and independence, they thrive in the security of a safe and structured environment. We discussed ways in which Mrs. Castillo could recognize when she was growing irritable with Michael and use it as a cue to begin giving three strikes.

Mrs. Castillo also brought up a common issue for parents: how to address their children's behavior, especially tantrums, in public places. Michael had a tantrum on the bus the previous week when his mother forgot to let him insert the Metrocard. He began screaming and crying until Ms. Castillo, mortified, got off the bus at the next stop, and walked the rest of the way home instead. I commended mother on her instincts and discussed how the natural consequence of walking home may have impacted Michael. We also reviewed additional strategies for helping Michael understand expectations during trips on the bus or errands to the grocery store in advance, and how to reinforce and support his behaviors during these outings.

I invited the Castillos to reflect on their initial concerns that Michael had ADHD and fears that he would be a "behavior problem" for a long time. They appeared to be as proud as Michael had been, leaving his time out and returning to the toys. We discussed how crucial it was to remain calm and self-regulated when trying to teach a child how to calm down and self-regulate. Of course, we laughed, how can you teach a child to calm down when you are yelling all the time? Mr. and Mrs. Castillo never had to put a bell on Michael's door, to alert them when he was up at night, as his nighttime adventures had stopped. I encouraged them to reach out to school to discuss Michael's improvements and to make sure the strategies used in both locations were consistent. We scheduled another follow-up appointment in a month to check in on Michael's progress, and to use as a booster session, if needed.

In many ways, the interventions which helped Michael dramatically change his behavior were quite basic and similar to what any clinician might use as part of a parent training protocol. The innovative component of this vignette is that it occurred in the pediatric clinic with a 3-year-old patient. Left untreated, it is very likely that Michael would have been kicked out of his daycare program, and perhaps diagnosed with Attention Deficit Hyperactivity Disorder or Oppositional Defiant Disorder by the time he reached elementary school. Michael's positive outcome is a testament to his parent's ability to easily access resources, their openness to changing their own behavior, and the importance of early identification and treatment.

Consult for Trauma

While most Healthy Steps consultations are related to concerns about children's challenging behaviors or developmental delays, having a clinically trained psychologist or social worker on site at a pediatric clinic can be useful for many difficulties faced by the families of very young children. Below is a vignette of a family seen at a clinic in the South Bronx, one of the poorest congressional districts in the nation, with the associated psychosocial stressors that often accompany living with poverty, including exposure to violence.

Dr. Kallowitz stopped by my office after seeing 2-week-old Sam and his mother. Dr. Kallowitz had known the family for 4 years, since the birth of Bella, Sam's older sister. While she had few concerns about the family in general, Dr. Kallowitz wanted to refer the family to Healthy Steps because of something that Erica, Sam and Bella's mother, had revealed at the visit. Dr. Kallowitz had casually asked about how Andre, the children's father, was doing, and Erica shared that he was recovering from a gunshot wound, and was only recently able to return to work.

Erica and Andre had been together for 7 years, and moved in together, with Andre's mother, Jessica, when Erica became pregnant with Bella. Erica was willing to speak with me and share the details of what had happened with Andre on the night that she delivered Sam. She explained that she had been taken to the hospital following a scheduled visit with her obstetrician. She was not due for another week, but was not surprised to learn that she was having contractions. She called Andre to let him know to meet her at the hospital. Andre left work and called his mother to share the exciting news. Andre explained that he was on his way home to pick up Erica's already packed hospital bag. Jessica, in turn, was eager to let Bella know that her baby brother was on his way. In their enthusiasm, Bella and Jessica waited by the window and watched for Andre to come running into the building. As Andre was running in, however, an argument erupted between a group of men near the building, and both Bella and Jessica heard the gunshot and Andre's cry of pain as the bullet hit his shoulder. The other men scattered, and Andre went up the stairs to see his family. Andre was ultimately taken to a different hospital from Erica, but was released and was able to make it to the delivery room before his son was born.

Despite the challenges prior to Sam's birth, Erica described an easy delivery and explained that she was glad to be back home with her family. She shared that Andre's wound was not serious. She was, however, concerned about Bella, who had clearly witnessed something terrifying. She explained that Bella seemed to want to share her memories of the shooting, asked many questions over and over again, and refused to go back to preschool. However, she was not having nightmares, had not developed any new fears, and had not demonstrated any regressive behavior. Erica explained that they tried to distract Bella from her focus on the shooting, hoping she would forget about it as soon as possible.

When I met with Erica and Bella later that week, Bella walked into my office with a smile on her face, eager to play with the toys provided, and to share her disappointment that Sam was not quite the playmate she had expected. She also told me that her father had "a boo boo" on his shoulder, but that it was getting better.

I enrolled the family in Intensive Services, and in addition, met with them several times over the next 2 months to address the concerns about Bella. Andre was not able to attend sessions because of his work schedule, though Erica regularly brought his questions to our appointments.

During these sessions we spoke about the importance of continuing to allow Bella the space to ask questions and speak of her experiences about the shooting, and the language to use in answering her questions in a developmentally appropriate manner, including the use of "feeling words." I also stressed the importance of communicating to Bella that, even though something scary happened, it was her family's job to keep her safe. I explained that maintaining routines and schedules was important in helping Bella both adjust to the birth of her baby brother and to reestablish a sense of security following the traumatic event. With this in mind, we were able to develop a plan to help Bella return to preschool.

I encouraged the family to pay attention to any changes in behavior, and explained that difficulties could arise at later points in development. Over the next year, Erica checked in with me when she brought the children for their medical appointments. Bella continued to do well, and, when I last saw the family before they moved out of the neighborhood, she was a highly articulate and playful kindergartner.

We include this example because it conveys a critical point in our work with families: while we cannot directly change the community in which they live, supporting parents to provide a warm, nurturing, and safe space in which children can grow impacts how children respond to the challenges and stressors of their everyday and potentially toxic environment. Erica and Andre's response to Bella's worries determined how she was able to interpret it, and supported the development of coping skills and self-regulation. Indeed, stressful events only become "toxic" for young children when they are unmitigated by caregivers.

Parental Mental Health

The following is a description of Parental Mental Health services, a therapeutic intervention based on the idea that supporting the mental health of the parent is critical for the well-being of the child. Integrating therapy services into primary care significantly reduces the multiple barriers that prevent many patients from accepting mental health treatment. New parents visit pediatric practices more frequently than they do any other medical facility, making it an ideal, yet often overlooked, venue in which to deliver services.

Leilani and her parents enrolled in Healthy Steps following her 2-month well-baby checkup with the pediatrician. At that early time in our program, the only enrollment criteria (due to a research protocol) were to be a first-time parent and to speak English. Leilani's mother, Susan, denied any history of childhood trauma. Susan and Abdul, in their early 20s, were eager to nurture their newborn, attended every appointment together, and discussed their experiences of being first-time parents. Susan and Leilani lived with her parents and brothers, and although Susan's parents did not approve of Abdul, he visited frequently.

At each visit, I provided anticipatory guidance and screened the parents for depression and anxiety. While neither parent reported symptoms or history of mental illness, we recognize that the birth of a child is a stressful life event, and strive to constantly assess parental well-being. As Leilani grew, I addressed the concerns of many first-time parents, including sleep training, managing tantrums, and picky eating. Abdul stopped attending pediatric appointments after Leilani's 18-month-visit, and Susan reported that although she and Abdul were no longer romantically involved, Leilani continued to see her father and his family on the weekends.

During Leilani's 30-month checkup, Susan reported being diagnosed with panic attacks following a few visits to the emergency room in the last month. She had already met with a psychiatrist, but expressed reluctance about using medication or talking about her personal life with a stranger. When I suggested that I could start seeing her to address these concerns, she was willing, as she reported that she felt she knew me well already. At her first therapy session, Susan explained, with pressured speech and tangential thoughts, that she did not believe her diagnosis of Panic Disorder was accurate, and that she was convinced that she had an undiagnosed cardiac problem. She was so confident that she was going to have a heart attack, she feared traveling to work by subway, and therefore missed shifts frequently. This in turn led to the very realistic fear that she could lose her job. Susan explained that she could not predict what triggered these episodes of chest pain, shortness of breath, racing heart, and sweating, and, therefore, never knew when the next one would strike. She was terrified that if she died, her daughter would be left alone.

I began by reviewing the symptoms of panic attacks and providing psycho-education on Panic Disorder. Although she could not imagine why she would be having panic attacks when she had no reason to be anxious, she acknowledged that her symptoms met the diagnostic criteria. She was relieved to learn she could meet with a psychiatrist on site at our clinic. In addition, attending sessions with the psychiatrist and myself on the same day made scheduling work shifts and child care arrangements easier.

Despite her initial ambivalence about her diagnosis, Susan embraced therapy and was open to talking about her feelings and experiences during our sessions. She also began to talk about our sessions with her family at home and soon learned that multiple family members, including her mother and aunt, also struggled with anxiety. Susan took pride in knowing that, unlike her family members, she addressed her symptoms directly and openly, something she hoped to teach her daughter to do as well. When we talked about the importance of recognizing warning signs of panic attacks and practicing relaxation techniques, she shared that with her family as well. As her confidence in therapy grew, Susan reported that she also noticed that she was more patient with Leilani, and more responsive to her needs, as she was less preoccupied with her fear of panic attacks.

Importantly, Susan also began to describe the dysfunctional relationship she had with Abdul. She voiced anger at his inconsistent and unreliable visits with Leilani, despite his not working or having any conflicting commitments, and her resentment that he did not contribute financially to her care. She casually mentioned that he screamed obscenities at her and sent her denigrating text messages in response to her requests to schedule the visits Leilani always asked for. I was struck by the fact that, even though I had been working with Susan for almost 3 years, this was the first time that she mentioned this abusive behavior to me. Susan was surprised when I suggested that these threats could be triggers of her panic attacks. In fact, she denied that Abdul's threats scared her, and was convinced that he would never actually hurt her. As we explored this further, however she slowly acknowledged how disturbed she was by Abdul's treatment of her and how his behavior (both his inconsistent caregiving for Leilani and his explosive temper) was affecting Leilani. While Susan noted defensively that she tried hard not to argue in front of Leilani, she acknowledged that their fights over the phone and texts were so upsetting that Leilani was clearly aware of the situation. Susan began to connect her symptoms of anxiety to earlier arguments with Abdul. By this point, she had shared so much of her treatment with her family members, that they began to coach her to hang up the phone when they noticed her getting upset on a call, or reminded her to breathe, a strategy we had first practiced in session, when she became agitated and began to pace following one of these conversations.

Susan continued in therapy for 10 months. She arranged for family members to watch Leilani for many of the sessions, so that she would be free to speak openly, and loudly, to express herself fully. She was gratified as her panic attacks grew less frequent and she gained confidence in both recognizing her symptoms of anxiety and using relaxation techniques to keep the most severe symptoms at bay. We established rules for safe communication with Abdul, and plans for how she could respond when his anger began to escalate. Medication helped initially, and she worked with the psychiatrist to gradually wean herself off, as she began to feel more capable of coping with her anxiety. She recognized that her new ability to regulate her affect helped her see choices in her behavior and gave her much more control over her life. The more control she felt over her life, the less she felt like a victim of Abdul's moods. As she reflected on her progress, Susan voiced confidence that Leilani was learning an important lesson too; she would never keep her daughter from her father, but she would not tolerate being mistreated by him or anyone. Susan's pride in mastering her symptoms was as strong as her initial panic regarding her mortality, and she began to date for the first time, and earned recognition for excellent work on the job.

Over the course of her treatment, not only did Susan conquer her debilitating symptoms, she also gained great insight about herself and her relationship with Abdul, lessons that both she and her daughter would most certainly benefit from. Seeking care in the pediatric clinic allowed her to begin treatment from a trusted provider quickly and conveniently and reduced the risk of her symptoms continuing untreated, an outcome that would have had significant personal and economic impact on her entire family.

Integrating mental health professionals, with a background in early childhood development, attachment theory, and the deleterious impact of trauma and toxic stress in primary pediatric practices is an efficient and cost-effective strategy for providing evidence-based care to the greatest number of families. Patients and their families can seek care in a convenient and non-stigmatizing environment and pediatricians are freed from addressing presenting problems beyond their expertise. Healthy Steps Specialists are able to identify vulnerable families and at risk children, and intervene early, supporting parents' abilities to build trusting and responsive relationships with their infants and young children. Providing therapy and psychiatric services for parents within the pediatric setting further increases the chances that families will get the intensive mental health services they need. Healthy Steps Specialists have the unique opportunity to work to prevent the transmission of multigenerational trauma and promote secure attachments, which buffer those most susceptible to the impact of toxic stress.

Reference

Felitti, V.J., Anda, R.F., Nordenberg, D., Williamson, D.F., Spitz, A.M., Edwards, V., Koss, M.P., Marks, J.S. (1998). The relationship of adult health status to childhood abuse and household dysfunction. *American Journal of Preventive Medicine, 14*(2), 45–258.

Index

© Springer International Publishing Switzerland 2016
R.D. Briggs (ed.), *Integrated Early Childhood Behavioral Health in Primary Care*, DOI 10.1007/978-3-319-31815-8

CPSIA information can be obtained
at www.ICGtesting.com
Printed in the USA
BVOW06*0223011116
466581BV00003B/5/P